Multiple Sclerosis

A GUIDE FOR THE NEWLY DIAGNOSED

Third Edition

Multiple Sclerosis

A GUIDE FOR THE NEWLY DIAGNOSED

Third Edition

Nancy J. Holland, EdD, RN, MSCN
Vice President, Clinical Programs
National Multiple Sclerosis Society
New York, New York

T. Jock Murray, MD
Dalhousie Multiple Sclerosis Research Unit
Halifax, Nova Scotia

Stephen C. Reingold, PhD
President
Scientific and Clinical Review Associates, LLC
New York, New York

Visit our website at www.demosmedpub.com

Library of Congress Cataloging-in-Publication Data

Holland, Nancy J.
  Multiple sclerosis : a guide for the newly diagnosed / Nancy J. Holland, T. Jock Murray, Stephen C. Reingold. – 3rd ed.
          p. cm.
  Includes bibliographical references and index.
  ISBN–13: 978–1–932603–27–9 (pbk. : alk. paper)
  ISBN–10: 1–932603–27–1 (pbk. : alk. paper)
1. Multiple sclerosis--Popular works.   I. Murray, T. J. II. Reingold, Stephen Charles, 1948- III. Title.
  [DNLM: 1. Multiple Sclerosis. WL 360 S299m 2007]
  RC377.H65 2007
  616.8'34--dc22

                                                        2006035632

Special discounts on bulk quantities of Demos Medical Publishing books are available to corporations, professional associations, pharmaceutical companies, health care organizations, and other qualifying groups. For details, please contact:

Special Sales Department
Demos Medical Publishing
386 Park Avenue South, Suite 301
New York, NY 10016
Phone: 800–532–8663 or 212–683–0072
Fax: 212–683–0118
Email: orderdept@demosmedpub.com

Made in the United States of America
07 08 09 10   5 4 3 2 1

Dedication

Those diagnosed with multiple sclerosis today owe a great debt of gratitude to Labe C. Scheinberg, MD. He opposed the voices who proclaimed defeat when faced with a diagnosis of multiple sclerosis, and insisted that much could be done to promote a productive and satisfying life, while limiting the negative impact of the disease.

Dr. Scheinberg was the champion of those with MS, from diagnosis throughout the disease course, during his lifetime. He was the inspirational leader whose vision shaped this book.

Acknowledgments

Special thanks to several staff members of the National Multiple Sclerosis Society for their input and assistance with the updating of this third edition: Nancy Law, Cristina Lipka, Stephen Nissen, Beverly Noyes, PhD, Ann Palmer, and Alicia Soto.

Thanks also to Jon Temme of the MS Society of Canada, to our consultant, Dr. Diana M. Schneider, and editor, Edith Barry, for their support throughout this project, and to the staff at Demos Medical Publishing.

Contents

Foreword

The diagnosis of multiple sclerosis (MS) is often accompanied by a perception that life has become unpredictable and uncontrollable. Obtaining authoritative and accurate information about the disease and its management is the first step to regaining emotional balance and the feelings of control and empowerment.

As with many medical issues, the problem is *finding* such information. The Internet is full of information that is often misleading at best and totally false at worst, and the literature is full of material on "cures" and treatments that lack validity.

The third edition of *Multiple Sclerosis: A Guide for the Newly Diagnosed* provides information that is both substantive and accurate. It has been developed by MS professionals with many years of experience in managing the disease, and is written with a straightforward and honest approach that provides all the information you need to begin to deal with this disease.

This is a new era in MS treatment. At no time previously have there been more ways to slow the disease process and manage its symptoms. The authors explore all of these in language that is understandable. They also recognize that there is a person behind the disease, and discuss topics such as choosing a health care provider and how to discuss MS with an employer. Things are changing so fast on the MS scene that one needs to keep up so as not to be left behind. While this book is written for the newly diagnosed, it clearly will also assist those previously diagnosed or simply interested in the latest information. I am proud to congratulate the authors on this excellent book!

Randall T. Schapiro, MD
The Schapiro Center for Multiple Sclerosis at
The Minneapolis Clinic of Neurology
and
Clinical Professor of Neurology
University of Minnesota
Minneapolis, Minnesota

Multiple Sclerosis

A GUIDE FOR THE NEWLY DIAGNOSED

Third Edition

1

||||||||||||||||||||||||||||||||||||||||||||||||||||||||||||||||||||||||||||||||||||||||||||||||||||||||||

What Is Multiple Sclerosis and How Is It Diagnosed?

It had been known for centuries that conditions involving the nervous system could cause progressive weakness. By the 19th century, physicians and pathologists recognized a particular disorder of young adults that was associated with scattered patches of scarring in the central nervous system (CNS)—the brain, spinal cord, and optic nerves. The neurologist who made the disease known in 1868 by clarifying its clinical and pathologic features, and gave the disease a name, was Jean Martin Charcot at the Hôpital Salpétrière in Paris. He described multiple sclerosis (MS) and its damage (lesions or plaques) in the brain, spinal cord, and optic nerves in relation to the symptoms that separate MS from other diseases. He named the disease "sclérose en plaques," the name still used for MS in French-speaking countries.

The modern name *multiple sclerosis* comes from the "sclerosed" or hardened plaques of scar tissue located at "multiple" sites throughout the CNS. Nerve fibers (axons) in the CNS are covered with a *myelin sheath*, which provides an insulating function similar to that

1

of the insulation around electrical wires. This insulation allows nerve conduction to proceed smoothly and at a rapid rate. Plaques or patches of inflammation damage the myelin around the nerve and disrupt the transmission of messages that communicate the desired action from the brain through the spinal cord to various parts of the body. For example, plaques that disrupt nerve fibers in the brain going to the legs could affect the ability to walk. Patients with multiple sclerosis often have a clinical history of episodes of neurologic symptoms that are related to multiple patches of inflammation in the spinal cord, brain, and optic nerves.

Under the microscope, the lesions or plaques are seen as areas in which there is a preponderance of thickly myelinated fibers, the *white matter* of the brain, so called because it appears pale due to the presence of myelin, compared to the *gray matter* in which there is little myelin. The area of plaque shows disruption of the myelin and some damage or loss of axons as well. There is an inflammatory reaction in these plaques, with some repair of fibers in older plaques and some scarring in very old plaques. More episodes of demyelination and more plaques may appear as years pass. Myelin can be repaired, allowing function to be restored, but conduction may be slower in these repaired fibers. Although repair can occur and may often be almost complete, the repeated myelin breakdown, incomplete repair, and accumulation of scarring lead to some progression of symptoms and signs of the disease after many years in most people with MS.

Once the disease was described and had a name, it was possible for physicians everywhere to recognize it. It became clear that MS was not uncommon, but was in fact the most common serious neurologic disease in young adults. It followed a number of different patterns and courses, sometimes appearing more than once in the same family, and was more common in certain parts of the world and in white people.

As the physicians and researchers of today seek answers and learn more about MS, they uncover more questions and more things to learn. But they are learning more, and there are more researchers working to find the cause and cure of MS, and more research dollars are being directed to this effort than ever before.

What Happens in Attacks of MS?

MS is defined as a neurologic disorder characterized by scattered plaques of demyelination throughout the white matter of the central nervous system. Let us look in more detail at what those terms mean.

The multiple scars that give the disease its name are the end result of the patchy breakdown of the insulating myelin cover that surrounds nerves. Although the symptoms (numbness in a limb, blurred vision in one eye, or weakness in a leg) may suggest that one plaque has developed, there probably is more than one, and possibly many. More surprisingly, some plaques may develop and heal without causing any symptoms.

At first there is an inflammatory response in the plaque, with cells present that are often seen in immunologic reactions. This has led to the belief that the episode of demyelination, or *attack*, may be an immunologic reaction of the body to some material in the myelin sheath, such as a protein (see Chapter 2). Why this happens is not certain. We know of other conditions in which the body's normal defense mechanism that reacts to "foreign" material seems to regard the normal proteins of the body as foreign and reacts against them.

When the episode of demyelination is settling down, other cells clean away the debris and remyelination, or repair of myelin, begins. As a result, the symptoms that occurred during the episode of demyelination may improve or completely disappear, although some lingering damage may have resulted. However, the new myelin conducts nerve impulses somewhat more slowly than normal unaffected myelin. If a physician tests the speed of conduction in these nerves, it may be slower than normal nerves. This change has been used as the basis for tests to look for evidence of nerve damage, such as visual evoked potentials, brain stem auditory evoked potentials, and sensory evoked potentials. These electrodiagnostic tests measure the time intervals for a message, such as light seen by the eye, to pass from the eye to the brain.

Episodes of demyelination accompanied by symptoms of MS may occur over many years. This is another hallmark of the disease—plaques that occur not only in multiple areas of the central nervous system but also in multiple events over time.

The Course of Multiple Sclerosis

The course of MS varies from person to person. We do not know why one person has a progressive course of symptoms and problems, while another has mild disease that produces little disability over time. Multiple sclerosis can have different patterns in people in the same family, and what pattern a person has seems to have nothing to do with anything we can measure in the body, life activities, or whatever steps are taken to manage the disease.

Despite this unpredictability, the courses of MS have been classified into four basic patterns defined by an international survey of MS experts:

Relapsing-Remitting—This form of MS is characterized by clearly defined acute attacks followed either by full recovery or by partial recovery but with some remaining symptoms. The periods between disease relapses are characterized by a lack of new symptoms, although the underlying disease process may be continuing. About 85 percent of patients with MS begin with this pattern.

The term *benign* is used to refer to a small number of people with relapsing-remitting MS who have a mild form of the disease and who remain fully functional in all neurologic systems 15 years after disease onset. This is the most difficult form of MS to "label" because it requires many years to identify this pattern. Many people with this form of the disease have mostly sensory symptoms. Because it cannot be reliably predicted early, treatment decisions are not based on the possibility that this course may occur.

Secondary Progressive—The disease pattern begins with a relapsing-remitting course. Within 10 to 15 years, approximately 50 percent of those with a relapsing-remitting course will enter a progressive phase, with a slow but steady worsening in overall condition. Patients may continue to have less frequent acute attacks or may stop having attacks altogether. It is not yet known whether treatment with one of the immunomodulating agents will decrease the number of people who develop this form of the disease, but that is the hope.

Primary Progressive—In this form of MS, the disease shows slow progression from its onset, without attacks but sometimes with occasional plateaus and temporary minor improvements. This form of MS is more commonly seen in people who develop the disease after the age of 40, and more often in men. About 15 percent of people with MS are initially diagnosed with this course.

Progressive-Relapsing—This pattern of MS shows progression from onset, but later on one or more attacks occur.

Remissions can occur at any time in the course of MS and can last for months or for many years. Why they occur is not known, and we are not able to tell in whom they will occur or when. Remissions are more common in the early stages of the disease and in the relapsing-remitting type. Plateaus in the course, with long periods when little change is seen in the affected person's symptoms is quite common.

The Diagnosis of Multiple Sclerosis

MS can be a difficult diagnosis to make. Although many patients who consult a neurologist can be diagnosed clinically without any doubt on the first visit, other situations are more difficult, especially when a patient has minor complaints, shows no "findings" or abnormalities on examination, or has a symptom—such as numbness—that also is common in many other conditions.

The diagnosis of MS is made by a physician, usually a neurologist, who takes a detailed history of the patient's symptoms and complaints, followed by a thorough physical and neurologic examination. Although the disease is suspected and ultimately diagnosed by the clinician's diagnostic skills, two things can assist in the diagnostic process.

The first is a set of criteria for establishing the diagnosis, which were developed in 2001 by the International Panel on the Diagnosis of Multiple Sclerosis, supported by the National Multiple Sclerosis Society and the International Federation of Multiple Sclerosis Societies, and modified in 2005 (Table 1-1). Although the terms may sound very general, the patient suspected of having MS is classified by the physician as having "possible" MS or "definite" MS. When a neurologist says that a person has MS, it means that he or she has had more than one episode or attack of symptoms occurring in multiple areas of the white matter of the CNS; in some instances, instead of attacks, there will have been progression over a long time, again characterized by changes typical of involvement of many areas of the white matter in the CNS.

When a person does not demonstrate all the criteria for MS, he or she may be classified as having possible MS on the basis that other conditions that might cause similar symptoms have been determined as being unlikely, and additional features of the disease may become evident in time. Common examples of patients who are initially classified as having possible MS are those who present with their first symptom (thus, there have not been multiple episodes and they have not been progressive over a long time) or those who have had repeated episodes but always in one site (thus, not multiple in the areas involved).

The second helpful aid to the neurologist is a group of tests that may confirm the suspicion of MS. Remember, though, that the diagnosis is still a clinical decision, and there is no test that says

TABLE 1-1 DIAGNOSTIC CRITERIA

Evidence of more than one area of CNS (central nervous system) involvement (dissemination in "space") and CNS involvement at more than one time (dissemination in "time") are required for a diagnosis of MS

||||||||||||||||||||||||||||||||||||||||||||||||||||||||||||||||||||||||||||||||||||||||||||||||||||||||||||||||||

CLINICAL PRESENTATION	ADDITIONAL DATA NEEDED FOR MS DIAGNOSIS
Two or more attacks; objective clinical evidence of two or more lesions in the central nervous system (CNS)	None
Two or more attacks; objective clinical evidence of one lesion in the CNS	Dissemination in space, demonstrated by: • Magnetic resonance imaging (MRI) *or* • Two or more MRI detected lesions consistent with MS plus positive cerebrospinal fluid (CSF) *or* • Await further clinical attack implicating a different site
One attack; objective clinical evidence of two or more lesions	Dissemination in time, demonstrated by: • MRI *or* • Second clinical attack
One attack; objective clinical evidence of one lesion (monosymptomatic presentation; clinically isolated syndrome)	Dissemination in space, demonstrated by: • MRI *or* • two or more MRI-detected lesions • consistent with MS plus positive CSF *and* Dissemination in time, demonstrated by: • MRI *or* • Second clinical attack

(Continued)

TABLE 1-1   (Continued)

||||||||||||||||||||||||||||||||||||||||||||||||||||||||||||||||||||||||||||||||||||||||||||||||||||||||||||

CLINICAL PRESENTATION	ADDITIONAL DATA NEEDED FOR MS DIAGNOSIS
Insidious neurologic progression suggestive of MS	One year of disease progression (retrospectively or prospectively determined) *and* Two of three of the following: 1. Positive brain MRI (nine T2 lesions or four or more T2 lesions with positive visual evoked potentials; 2. Positive spinal cord MRI (two or more focal T2 lesions); 3. Positive CSF

Adapted from McDonald et al. Recommended diagnostic criteria for MS. *Ann Neurol* 2001; 50:121–127 and Polman et al. 2005 Revisions to the McDonald diagnostic criteria. *Ann Neurol* 2005;58:840–846.

definitively that MS is present. The test can only suggest changes that are compatible with the diagnosis, and the neurologist uses this to aid his or her clinical judgment.

Clinical Examination

The clinical examination has three major parts: history, examination, and tests.

History

The history includes not only the story of your symptoms and complaints but also your general health during your lifetime, your operations and accidents, illnesses in your family, occupational information, and other details. This often is the most important part of the examination. The neurologist often makes the diagnosis during this part of the assessment, even before the neurologic examination or diagnostic tests, which are most often used to confirm the neurologist's suspicions from the history.

Examination

To get a complete picture of your health and to better under-stand your symptoms, the neurologist performs a general physical examination that includes listening to your chest and heart, taking your blood pressure, and examining your muscles and skin, as well as a neurologic examination that includes examining your eyes, the cranial nerves to your head and face, your strength, sensation, and ability to detect vibration over various parts of the body, your reflexes, and your balance and walking. Sometimes a patient is surprised to have his or her feet and abdomen examined when the complaint is of numbness in a hand. However, this overall examination provides a picture of your nervous system and is able to identify other condi-tions that might explain the symptoms you are experiencing.

Tests

A number of tests can help to confirm that MS may be present and also can identify other problems that mimic its symptoms. Some patients so clearly have MS when they are assessed that no tests are necessary, or only one test may be used to confirm the disease and rule out other problems that might be under suspicion. The follow-ing are only the most commonly used and valuable tests.

MAGNETIC RESONANCE IMAGING (MRI) A few decades ago, MRI would have seemed like science fiction—a test that pro-duces a picture of your brain as you lie inside a huge electromagnet that momentarily spins the molecules in your body. Minutes later, the computer produces a remarkable picture of your nervous system that looks much like a black and white photograph from an anatomy textbook. More remarkable for those who care for people with MS, the MRI is particularly good at detecting the patchy areas of change in the nervous system that occur with the disease. It has become the most accurate and helpful test for MS; it is positive for changes consistent with the disease in 9 of 10 people with proven MS.

The MRI examination is done while you lie on a table that moves inside a tube-like space in a large machine that holds a magnet. You will need to lie very still while the magnet sends information to a computer that receives thousands of tiny bits of information and uses them to generate pictures. These images are like slices or views at many levels throughout the brain or the spinal cord, or wherever the scanner is set. Often, a dye or contrast material (gadolinium) is injected into a vein to obtain more detailed pictures.

No discomfort is associated with the procedure, and the scanners are becoming faster, so that the length of time for a scan decreases each year. Some people have some feeling of claustrophobia and dislike the closed in feeling of the narrow space and the noise the machine makes. Most people can tolerate it well, especially when they know how important it is and when they have received a clear explanation of the procedure and receive support and encouragement from the staff. However, the anxiety experienced by some people can be easily reduced by mild sedation, such as diazepam (Valium®) 10 mg taken prior to the MRI. You need to ask your doctor for a prescription for Valium at the time he or she requests the test. MRI is an amazing technologic advance that can help in the diagnosis of many diseases and also is helpful in research. However, there are some drawbacks to its completeness as a test for MS. Because it is so complex, the machinery, support systems, and personnel needed to operate them are very expensive. The cost of the test often is in the range of $500 to over $1,000—higher if more complex procedures are necessary.

Another drawback is that the MRI is not always positive or conclusive in patients with MS, especially if they are at an early stage in the disease and have had only a few or very mild symptoms. Furthermore, the test does not "show MS"; it shows changes that *could be* due to MS. We must remember that other conditions occasionally cause similar changes. That is why the clinical picture is most helpful and can indicate whether other problems should be considered or whether this is a typical story of MS symptoms, with typical findings of MS on examination, and with typical changes in keeping with MS on the MRI.

Finally, although the MRI can confirm the diagnosis, it does not tell us all the things you and we want to know, such as whether the disease is mild or advanced or whether it is getting worse (those are clinical features). Further developments in MRI techniques undoubtedly will allow us to answer many more of these questions.

CEREBROSPINAL FLUID The cerebrospinal fluid (CSF) surrounds the brain and spinal cord and fills some cavities within the central nervous system. A fine needle can be inserted into the lower back (below the end of the spinal cord) to remove a sample of this clear fluid for examination of cells, protein, and electrolytes; this is a lumbar puncture, which is also called an LP or a spinal tap.

A number of tests can be done on the CSF fluid, but the most useful in MS is to examine the proteins for the presence of *oligoclonal bands*; the fluid is put on a gel and an electrical current is passed through it in the laboratory to separate its protein contents into these bands. Approximately 9 of 10 people who have a well-established pattern of MS have bands in the CSF, but unfortunately this pattern is less common in early and very mild cases. The CSF is usually examined if the MRI is not conclusive but the clinical picture is suggestive of MS. It is also an important test if the pattern of involvement is primary progressive MS to verify that the progressive disease is really MS.

Many people have heard that having a lumbar puncture is uncomfortable, but it usually does not cause much discomfort and can be done on an outpatient basis. Unfortunately, about one-third of people get a headache when they sit up after the test, a problem that may last for days. Lying flat on the abdomen to facilitate closure of the puncture site and taking abundant oral fluids to replace CSF lost through testing should minimize this side effect.

EVOKED POTENTIAL STUDIES The principle of evoked potential (EP) studies is simple. Nerves that have experienced demyelination conduct impulses more slowly than normal, even if they have healed and remyelinated. Evoked potential studies measure the rate and form of the impulse as it passes through specific nerves. The only evoked potential study that can strongly support the diagnosis of MS is the visual study.

Visual evoked potential studies assess the conduction of messages through the optic nerves behind the eyes. To stimulate the visual system, the person may be asked to watch a TV screen that shows a checkerboard or some other pattern that rapidly changes, producing a stimulus that passes through the visual system to the occipital cortex of the brain (located at the back of the skull) where vision is processed. Electrodes over the scalp measure the wave form and the speed of the impulse to determine whether one differs from the other or if characteristic changes consistent with a diagnosis of MS are present.

The visual evoked potential study is most useful if there is evidence of neurologic involvement in an area other than the visual system, and the neurologist is seeking involvement in another area; in this case, the optic nerve. If the person has a history of a definite optic neuritis, the test is of less value, as it is already known that the optic nerve is affected.

Watchful Waiting

Uncertainty is difficult to cope with, and many people would like answers to their problems even if they are unpleasant. Unfortunately, definitive answers are not always possible.

In perhaps 10 to 15 percent of cases, the answer to the question "Is MS the cause of these symptoms?" remains uncertain even after all available examinations and tests have been done. By this time the neurologist will have eliminated other possibilities such as a tumor or a disc pressing on the nervous system. He or she often will know that MS could be causing the symptoms but that other conditions might also be responsible. This uncertainty can be upsetting, but the approach at this point must be one of "wait and see," with periodic examinations and visits to the physician if new problems appear or changes occur. In most instances, the diagnosis becomes clear over time. This requires patience by both the person with symptoms and the physician, but if they agree that they will wait together, the patient usually accepts the situation, having been reassured about the absence of tumors and other worries. In some instances, the problem later turns out to be something other than MS, often a mild, benign, or treatable condition. It is better to wait than to be prematurely labeled as having MS on the basis of unclear evidence.

The Outcome

When a person develops MS, she or he naturally wants to know what this will mean in the long term, relative to life, health, and family. Unfortunately, uncertainty and unpredictability are characteristics of the disease as well as of its pattern of symptoms and course. What we *can* say in general terms is that the outlook is improving year by year and will continue to improve. Even before there was therapy to treat the underlying disease, the life expectancy of most people with MS had been extended to within the normal range as a result of the development of treatments such as antibiotics for bladder and kidney infections and better therapy for many of the complications of the disease. Newly available treatments for the underlying cause of the disease undoubtedly will change the long-term tendency for repeated attacks, progression, and disability, but we still have a long way to go. Research is proceeding rapidly and although it will never be fast enough or great enough for those suffering daily with MS, we are heading in the right direction.

2

||||||||||||||||||||||||||||||||||||||||||||||||||||||||||||||||||||||||||||||||||||||||||||||||||||||||||||||||||||||||||||||

What Is the Cause
of Multiple Sclerosis?

Multiple sclerosis (MS) has been known and studied as a distinct disease since the mid-1800s. However, the cause of the disease (what scientists call the "etiology") remains unknown. Many theories abound as to the root cause of MS, but none has been proved. Because understanding what causes a disease can lead to a better sense of how to prevent and treat it, and because the cause of MS remains a mystery, research into its etiology is one of the most active areas of scientific exploration. Recent findings have brought us closer to an understanding of MS and have led to new therapies and new approaches for future treatments.

Theories About the Cause of MS

Multiple sclerosis appears—or, as clinicians say, "presents"— as a neurologic disease affecting the central nervous system (CNS: the brain, spinal cord, and optic nerves). In other words, signs and symptoms of the disease can be attributed to problems in nervous system function. Consequently, scientific work has focused on how nervous system problems in MS develop.

Autopsy studies of the bodies of individuals who had MS before death reveal the hallmarks of the disease in the CNS. This includes evidence of attack by the body's immune system, such as inflammation or swelling of tissue, breakdown and loss of white matter or myelin surrounding nerve fibers and of nerve fibers themselves, and the appearance of hardened scars where myelin has been lost. There may be many such scars—called lesions—widely distributed in the CNS, thus giving rise to the disease's English name, multiple (many) sclerosis (scars). Immune cells, such as T lymphocytes and macrophages—normally seen in the blood stream—are present in the lesions and are activated against CNS tissue. These facts related to immunology in MS have been extremely important because the CNS normally is immune "privileged" and immune cells usually remain in the bloodstream outside of the CNS. In MS, however, such cells become activated and are able to penetrate the barrier between the blood and the nervous system—the blood-brain barrier (BBB).

Penetration of activated immune cells across the BBB into the CNS triggers a further complex process of immune-mediated damage of myelin (primarily) and underlying nerve fibers. Myelin serves as a structural and electrical insulator around nerve fibers, and when it is damaged, and when nerve fibers themselves are damaged, this causes a disruption of the of electrical and chemical signals responsible for nerve conduction from the brain and spinal cord to muscles and from sensory organs back to the brain and spinal cord. When nerve signals become disrupted, uncoordinated, and even blocked by this immune-mediated damage, this brings about the typical neurologic problems in balance, gait, bladder and bowel control, numbness, pain, and other symptoms typical of MS.

Tissue Abnormalities, Infections, and the Environment: Links to an MS Cause?

Many theories have been explored as to why the myelin of the CNS is attacked by a person's own immune system in MS, a so-called "autoimmune" (self-immune) attack. For example, congenital defects in nervous system structure or function that might make myelin and nerve fibers vulnerable and more susceptible to immune attack have been considered. For many years, efforts to demonstrate that nervous system tissue might be abnormal in people who develop MS have been fruitless. In recent years, however, sophisticated magnetic resonance imaging studies have suggested that CNS white matter—the myelin that is a target of immune attack in MS—may in fact not be normal after all. So-called "normal-appearing" white matter (NAWM) in apparently intact and undamaged areas of the CNS may be subtly abnormal. This may indeed be a focus of vulnerability to immune attack. Whether an underlying structural defect in myelin can help cause MS, or whether such abnormalities in NAWM are a consequence rather than a cause of disease remains unclear. Investigations into the cause and meaning of NAWM in the CNS of people with MS are an important area of current research.

It has been speculated that MS is the result of a direct effect of infection with a virus or bacteria on nervous system myelin or that such infection can trigger an autoimmune attack. This has been an intensive area of MS research over the past half century. The speculation arose because some viral and bacterial infections can cause damage in the nervous system and do cause other nervous system diseases, such as poliomyelitis and bacterial meningitis, to name only a few. Multiple viruses and bacteria have been proposed to be linked to MS over the years, including measles virus, herpes viruses, hepatitis virus, chlamydial bacteria, and others, all of which have been associated with MS by one or more investigators over the years. However, none of these has ever been shown to be a cause of MS, and no single infectious agent has ever been unequivocally associated with development or worsening of the disease.

The possibility that an environmental toxin or even a dietary imbalance may be the cause of MS has been considered. Although toxic substances and diet can cause other nervous system problems, no research has supported such a direct cause for MS. Occasional reports have been made of "clusters" of MS, where more cases than might be expected are found in towns, neighborhoods, or even among individuals from the same school class. Such reports have triggered epidemiologic studies—and such studies are still being pursued—to determine if such clusters are real or simply coincidence; and if real, to evaluate any environmental factors that might be involved. None, to date, has shown a direct environmental agent to be involved in the development of MS.

In spite of years of investigation into infectious or environmental causes for MS, there have been little data to support either of these factors as a potential cause of the disease. However, claims still appear from time to time in the media or scientific literature of the "latest" cause of the disease, and generally upon further study, such claims have little merit. However, because a possible association between MS and such potential causes could be one of the unsolved mysteries of the disease, these areas are still being explored. Until the cause of MS is discovered, rational, careful studies in these areas are still appropriate.

A More Likely Possibility: Underlying Immune System Problems in MS

Research on the cause of MS since the mid-1950s has focused increasingly on the immune system function in MS and on the theory that MS is an autoimmune disease. Autoimmunity is by no means unique to MS. Diseases such as rheumatoid arthritis (RA), systemic lupus erythematosus (SLE), juvenile-onset, or type 1, diabetes (JD), scleroderma, myasthenia gravis, and others are also believed to be autoimmune in nature. Many of these diseases share some important characteristics. In each, cells and/or antibodies of a person's own immune system attack and destroy what appear to be normal tissues of a person's body. Most (but not all) such diseases share a tendency to be more prevalent in women than in men (juvenile-onset diabetes is an exception: gender distribution is about equal between men and women and, in a few rare conditions, male predominance is the rule). All may be susceptible to treatment through a variety of routes that suppress or otherwise regulate immune function.

The evidence that the immune system is involved in MS is fairly clear. First, people with MS seem to have clear-cut abnormalities in immune function compared with healthy individuals. These include, among other factors, evidence that specific white blood cells (T lymphocytes or T cells) are present in the CNS that are primed to "recognize" and launch attacks against tissues of the nervous system, such as myelin and nerve fibers. In individuals with MS, there is clear and specific reaction of white T cells against proteins that compose CNS myelin. Interestingly, it has been known since the mid-1990s that individuals *without* MS also have such T cells that can react against myelin, but in such individuals these cells remain circulating in the bloodstream, separated from the CNS by the blood-brain barrier (BBB). In MS, the BBB is broken or breached, allowing the immune cells to flow into the CNS tissue and initiate their damaging effects. Breaks in the BBB can actually be visualized with contrast-enhancing (gadolinium-enhanced) magnetic resonance images (MRI) and other sophisticated imaging techniques.

An additional clue to the immune system's role in MS is the overrepresentation of cells and other immune system components that enhance immune responses in individual with the disease— so-called proinflammatory immune cells—and a relative underrepresentation of cells and immune mediators that suppress immune responses—anti-inflammatory cells. Most notably, in tissue from individuals with MS, immune system cells are found in active lesions of the brain and spinal cord. These immune characteristics are not normally seen in individuals who do not have MS.

Although immune system involvement in MS seems clear, evidence that the problem is *autoimmune* is difficult to obtain in humans. Actual proof of autoimmunity requires that immune system cells that cause damage in one patient be injected into a different, healthy patient and cause damage and disease there as well. Although this kind of experiment can be done in laboratory animals to prove autoimmunity, it obviously is not ethical to undertake such studies using humans, since such experiments would cause autoimmune disease in otherwise healthy people. In laboratory animals with a disease called experimental allergic (or autoimmune) encephalomyelitis (EAE), which many consider to be a reasonably good research model for human MS, such experiments proving autoimmunity have been done. So, evidence of the autoimmune nature of MS in humans is largely indirect and has been extrapolated from studies on laboratory animals with MS-like EAE.

For this reason alone, EAE has proven to be a very fruitful animal disease model to help understand human MS. While EAE is not MS and laboratory animals are not humans, there are many similarities in clinical symptoms and CNS lesion patterns between EAE in laboratory animals and MS in humans. These similarities have led most investigators to conclude that EAE and MS have similar involvement of the immune system. EAE thus serves in many regards as a "model" for the study of MS, and in particular for studies on the very specific elements of immune function that might be involved in MS-like disease. EAE studies not only have contributed to our understanding of immune problems in MS but also have been used productively to demonstrate a "proof of concept" for new immune therapies that might be used for human MS; and EAE studies have led to some of the immune-modulating drugs that are used in MS today.

The Role of Genetics in MS

The possibility that MS may have a genetic component that underlies its cause has been known for decades, based primarily on the fact that the disease sometimes seems to "run" in families. We know that MS is not directly inherited, but it is increasingly clear that a complex set of genetic factors helps to determine who may be susceptible to MS and who may not. Observations that suggest a genetic factor in MS come from studies of many populations around the world.

First, approximately 20 percent of all individuals with MS have at least one additional family member, either in the same generation or in a different generation, who also has or had an MS diagnosis or symptoms that are characteristic of MS even if a diagnosis was never made. While more cases of MS appear to be sporadic (with no other known cases in the family), this 20 percent rate of *concordance* (the occurrence of disease in more than one family member) suggests a genetic link or genetic influence for many individuals who have the disease. However, the concordance rate among family members is in itself not high enough to prove a genetic link, certainly not high enough to support a direct disease inheritance and, in itself, does not help us understand which genes might be involved. Such concordance could happen, for example, simply because of a shared environmental cause or trigger for MS. However, results from a large-scale study in Canada in the 1990s indicated that the tendency for multiple cases of MS to occur in families is truly genetic and not due to any sort of shared environmental or dietary factor.

In "multiplex" families in which more than one case of MS may occur, the risk of disease is still quite low. In the United States, about one in 1,000 people have MS; when a family member (parent, sibling, aunt/uncle) already has the disease, the risk increases to 2 to 5 per 100, depending on the degree of relationship. This is an increase in susceptibility but still a relatively low risk. Important information also comes from the study of twins where only one or both have MS.

Among nonidentical ("fraternal" or dizygotic) twins, the risk for MS to occur in both twins resembles that for any other sibling (2 to 5 percent); however, in identical twins (monozygotic twins, who are genetically identical), the risk of both twins having MS if one twin has been diagnosed rises dramatically to as high as 30 percent, a clear indication of the importance of genetic factors.

Beyond the reasonably frequent occurrence of MS in more than one family member, it also has long been known that there are ethnic or religious populations in the world that are *genetically isolated*— they rarely or never marry or bear children outside their own group and thus have developed a relatively restricted and unique gene pool. MS never or rarely occurs in some of these groups. Examples include such religious sects as the Hutterites in Canada and such ethnic groups as Eastern European gypsies. While living in areas where there is a relatively high incidence of MS, these groups seem to be protected from MS. Such genetically isolated populations are of great interest in disease research—not only those that seem to be "resistant" but also those in which disease may be prevalent. Such populations most likely have a more restricted pool of genes, raising the possibility that they can be used to more easily isolate disease-relevant gene factors. Studies on genetics have been undertaken in genetically isolated populations in locations such as western Finland and Tasmania and are currently underway in Iceland where scientists hope that new clues to MS genetics may be easier to obtain.

Related to this is the fact that there are racial differences in the incidence and even in the clinical appearance of MS. In North America, the disease occurs more commonly among white people than among African Americans, even in the same community, and the clinical symptomatology and severity of the disease may be different in these two groups. And there may be differences in how individuals of different racial background respond to MS therapies as well. Pure African Bantus virtually never devlop MS, although whites living in the same part of Africa are susceptible. Importantly, genetic studies of African Americans with MS may yield important clues to MS genetics more generally. African Americans often have a mixed genetic background—a combination of original African ancestral genes and white genes that have been inherited through white ancestors since the time of slavery in North America. Through "admixture" analysis of the genetic background of African Americans with MS, Africans who do not have MS, and whites with MS, it may be possible to more closely identify MS disease-related genes, and such studies are under way. Finally, MS is seen much less often in Asians, and in a clinical type quite different from that of whites.

While in some cases, issues of racial or ethnic difference in MS may be simply due to problems of ascertainment (determining who has the disease in a population) or of differences in the nature of medical care, there seems to be good evidence that the same kinds of genetic factors that underlie racial and ethnic differences overall may also have an impact on diseases such as MS. All of these factors point to a clear genetic influence on MS even if the disease is not directly inherited.

While such information might one day provide us with the ability to predict susceptibility, it cannot yet help us. The risk rates are low even within families in which MS already exists. Inheritance patterns in MS are extremely complex and poorly understood. Large genetic studies to search for common genetic factors that might underlie MS have been undertaken in the United States, Canada, the United Kingdom, Europe, and Australia, taking advantage of the existence of families with multiple individuals who have MS. From these studies, we have learned that no single genetic factor is responsible for MS or even dominant in the MS genetic picture. Rather, there are many genetic factors that might contribute to MS susceptibility. There is no current identified single gene, and there is not likely to be one, that can be said to cause MS, as has been shown for diseases such as Huntington's chorea, Duchenne muscular dystrophy, and cystic fibrosis.

Genetic research in MS is among the most highly technologic in the field today. With each year, new findings are being made that benefit directly and immediately from scientific progress in human and animal genetics more generally. The description of the full human genome in the late 1990s helped to identify genes that make us "human" and set the stage for discovery of genes that might underlie specific human traits and specific human diseases. The human genome map has led to efforts in the first years of the 21st century to describe completely the human *haplotype* map—a description of the blocks of genes that tend to be inherited together from generation to generation. This so called "hap map" will greatly reduce the complexity of the search for disease-related genes in the human population. Application of these technologies to MS has been among the first disease-related studies to be undertaken.

However, MS is not just a genetic disease, and genetics cannot be the whole story in MS. The fact that identical twins are not always concordant for MS (since both twins have an MS diagnosis only about 30 percent of the time) clearly indicates that, as important as genetic factors may be, other nongenetic factors contribute to determining MS susceptibility.

What Sets Off the Disease? Possible Environmental Triggers

For decades, studies of where MS exists in the world and where it is absent ("epidemiology" and "demographics") have suggested that some triggering factor in the environment must start the disease process. Data suggest that such a factor—most likely infectious— must be encountered before the age of 15 in order for the disease process to be triggered later in life. Although somewhat controversial, this finding has stimulated the search over the half century for a virus or other infectious agent that causes, or at least triggers, MS.

Many common and uncommon viruses have been proposed as causative agents for MS over the past several decades. Many of these proposals have been based on the presence of virus in tissues from individuals with MS or, more often, the presence of immune system antibodies against viruses in the blood. In recent years, technology has become more sophisticated, and such searches include the use of polymerase chain reaction (PCR) analysis to detect protein "footprints" in blood, cerebrospinal fluid, and tissue even if whole virus cannot be seen. In each case in which claims for causative or triggering infectious agents have been made using such analyses, to date further scientific work needed to confirm and expand upon the original claim has failed to support the original claims. Ongoing work continues to focus on human herpesvirus 6 (HHV-6), a common virus that causes roseola in infants and has been linked by some scientists to MS. The Epstein-Barr virus (EBV), the cause of infectious mononucleosis, continues to attract attention as a possible trigger for MS. A common bacterium, *Chlamydia pneumoniae*, which is responsible for "walking pneumonia," also has been linked to MS by some researchers, but original claims of a causative or triggering link for this bacterium have not held up.

Rather than focusing on a single infectious agent, many scientists now believe that individuals with MS have a heightened immune antibody response against a host of common and uncommon viruses and other infectious agents, and that past claims based on antibody responses against viruses are likely very misleading. While this has not stopped the search for a specific MS agent, it has much of the ongoing research searching for an infectious agent, and any claims that have resulted have beeen subject to skepticism in recent years.

With a new understanding of the importance of immunology in the MS disease process, many scientists have shifted their view of the role of specific viruses and other infectious agents in MS away from the search for a direct cause of the disease toward learning how an immune system response against an infectious agent may result in a later autoimmune disease. Increased attention has been paid to the possibility that many viruses, bacteria, and perhaps other pathogens could serve as a trigger for the autoimmune process that becomes MS.

Demyelination: The Cause of Symptoms

The damage done by an immune reaction against myelin and nerve tissue in the CNS might truly be considered the cause of MS since it is this process that results in neurologic signs and symptoms observed in the clinic and experienced by the individual with MS. As noted previously, immune system T cells normally in the bloodstream become activated against components of brain myelin. They cross the barrier between the bloodstream and the CNS, causing local inflammation in the brain and spinal cord in scattered places, but most often around blood vessels and cavities in the brain called *ventricles.* This process eventually results in inflammation and damage to the myelin insulation around nerve fibers and may result in damage and loss of nerve fibers as well. Lost myelin is extremely difficult for the nervous system to repair, and soon cells called *astrocytes* form scars where myelin previously existed.

Inflammation, loss of myelin and nerve fibers, and subsequent scarring result in reduced conduction of nerve signals within the CNS, out to muscles, and back from sensory organs. These conduction problems produce the symptoms that characterize the disease.

So, What Is the Cause of MS?

Multiple sclerosis is, to be sure, a complex disease that is just beginning to be unraveled. There remains no known single cause of MS, and it is likely that the disease is the result of a number of related factors. While symptoms come from problems in the nervous system, MS appears to be a disease of immune system function, most likely an autoimmune disease, which attacks the central nervous system. Although the disease is not directly inherited, there is a genetic susceptibility. A triggering factor, or a combination of factors, seems to be involved, but no definite virus, bacterium, or other infectious or environmental agent has been identified. The ultimate consequence of the immune system problems in MS is the entrance of immune cells into the CNS, attack of myelin around nerve fibers, and eventual myelin and nerve fiber loss and scarring. The entire process results in the failure of nerve signals to operate properly, resulting in the well-known symptoms that are the hallmark of MS.

3

||||||||||||||||||||||||||||||||||||||||||||||||||||||||||||||||||||||||||||||||||||||||||||||||||||||||||||

What Treatment
Is Available?

Managing the medical aspects of treating multiple sclerosis (MS) is accomplished through a partnership of health professionals, the person with MS, and his or her family. In this chapter, we address both the symptomatic treatment and management of the disease course.

People often say that there is no treatment for a disease when what they really mean is that there is no "magic bullet," a simple cure that makes the disease go away, as penicillin may do for pneumonia. As with most medical diseases, there is yet no "cure" for MS, but there are many treatments and approaches that will help you to understand and cope with the challenges, as well as many ways to reduce its symptoms. Additionally, we are in an era in which there are agents that lessen the number and severity of attacks, the progression of the disease, and the development of disability.

Resources

One of the most important first steps in dealing with MS is to learn more about it. You need to know what you can do to stay healthy and to reduce the problems that may confront you and your family. You are in control of much that is important in managing this disease. The fact that you are reading this book shows that you are already taking charge of one of the first things over which you have control—being informed and educated about MS.

Although your physician and other health-care professionals will be able to offer many of the treatments and procedures discussed, you should begin by facilitating access to additional information through membership in the national (U.S.), Canadian, or other national MS Society. Some people are reluctant to join at first because they are uncertain of what commitment this might involve. There is none! Being a member will provide access to the best up-to-date information and help with issues and problems related to having MS. You can learn about ongoing research and important advances as they occur. MS societies and their local chapters have many pamphlets and educational programs on all important aspects of the disease (see Chapter 11).

There are many books about MS. Some are excellent, and others are not. Some are by professionals who manage the disease, some are by individuals who have successfully adapted to its limitations, and some are by enthusiasts who are proposing new treatments and often are selling them. Consulting the MS Society will help to keep a balanced view because the publications it recommends have been carefully reviewed for both accuracy and usefulness.

People with MS often hear of possible treatments from friends and the media, and it is often difficult to distinguish those that are useful from those that are not (or that may actually be harmful). We strongly recommend that you check any suggested treatments made by people other than your physician or nurse with reliable sources, including the Canadian or National Multiple Sclerosis Society or the books recommended in the Additional Readings section of this book.

Types of Treatment

Treatments in MS can be grouped into different categories:

- Management of the acute attack
- Treatment of the underlying disease
- Management of symptoms
- Interventions related to emotional and social issues

Management of Acute Attacks

When there is a change in symptoms over a few days or weeks, with the development of new symptoms or the worsening of old ones, the event may be a new "attack" of the disease. It usually means that new patches of inflammation and demyelination are occurring in either new or old sites in the central nervous system (CNS)—the brain, spinal cord, and optic nerves. These often are mild and cease after a few days or weeks. Treatment may be indicated if the symptoms are severe or continue to worsen. The swelling and inflammation in the plaques of demyelination can be reduced by high-dose intravenous (IV) steroids (methylprednisolone).

Some people may begin to recover soon after steroid therapy has started, but for others, improvement may occur only slowly, even weeks after the treatment. As some spontaneous recovery is expected after most acute attacks, it sometimes is difficult to know how much was due to the treatment and how much would have occurred without it.

Not all episodes of new symptoms require therapy with IV steroids, but a number of treatment schedules can be used if indicated. There are some differences in the total steroid dose, the number of days of treatment, and the time between doses, but all are characterized by a high dose over a short period. This usually is given on an outpatient basis and generally is well tolerated, although some people experience emotional changes during the therapy and may have trouble sleeping.

If there is numbness in a limb, dizziness, or some other symptom that is annoying but not limiting in any way, your neurologist may decide to wait and see if the problem clears spontaneously, as it often does. An attack that has stopped progressing and is improving may be allowed to clear on its own. High-dose steroids help people to recover from an attack somewhat faster, but since they might recover just as well with time, decisions about treatment must be made on an individual basis. The repetitive use of steroids can have long-term effects that include cataracts and osteoporosis; therefore, their use should be reserved for more serious attacks that are not clearing spontaneously. A rare but important complication is avascular necrosis of the hip which requires a hip replacement.

Although it is reasonable to rest when you have MS, especially during attacks, it generally is overdone and overrecommended. There is good evidence that you will be tired if you do not get a reasonable amount of rest (although some tiredness in MS, referred to as MS fatigue, does not respond to rest), but there is little evidence that your MS will be worse with less rest. The fear that MS will become worse if you do not rest is without foundation and makes people fearful of doing normal things when they have symptoms. People may rest too much and thereby feel weary and weak, or stop work or neglect their responsibilities when they are capable of continuing these activities. A reasonable approach is to rest when you are tired and to develop a schedule that allows for a slower pace. Learning to manage despite the fatigue is the best approach.

The best advice to people with MS is not "rest, with reasonable activity," but rather "stay active, with reasonable rest." The difference is in placement of the emphasis. Slow down and rest more when symptoms and fatigue are a problem or when an attack occurs, but stay as active as you can and increase your activity again when the symptoms are relieved.

Treatment of the Underlying Disease

We now have available therapies that offer the promise of having an impact on the ultimate course of the disease, with minimal side effects for most people. None of the currently available therapies will cure or completely stop the disease, but these medications can reduce the number and severity of attacks and result in less progression and disability over the years.

These therapies include two different interferon beta preparations, glatiramer acetate and natalizumab. They have been approved in many countries, and other agents will soon appear. These agents have been approved for use in MS based on extensive clinical trials. Most neurologists make their decision as to which drug is appropriate for a given patient based on that individual's disease characteristics and lifestyle.

Fairly good evidence indicates that the agents discussed in the following sections are helpful if they are used in the early relapsing stages of the disease, but evidence for their effectiveness if the disease changes to a progressive phase is unclear at this time.

It is important to recognize that these agents help, but do not stop, problems or changes caused by MS. Some people who have taken them have greater expectations than the treatments can deliver and become discouraged and stop the drugs because they continue to have further problems. The hope is that, over time, you will be better than if you did not have the treatment, not that you will suddenly notice yourself improving or even that relapses will cease completely.

DISEASE MANAGEMENT CONSENSUS STATEMENTS   Both the National Multiple Sclerosis Society of the United States and the Canadian MS Clinics Network have issued statements on the use of disease-modifying agents.

These consensus statements are education tools that are used to promote the approved disease-modifying therapies, for appropriate candidates, early in the disease course. The U.S. document also serves as a communication device for interactions with insurers at the local and national levels to insure access to these drugs across the various health insurance plans.

||||||||||||||||||||||||||||||||||||||||||||||||||||||||||||||||||||||||||||||||||||||||||||||||||||||||||||||||

NATIONAL MS SOCIETY INFORMATION SOURCEBOOK

www.nationalmssociety.org/sourcebook.asp

The National MS Society's
Disease Management Consensus Statement

SUMMARY

This document has not been updated to reflect the return of Tysabri to the market in 2006.

INTRODUCTION

The Consensus Statement is an education and advocacy tool that is used to promote increased access to the approved disease-modifying therapies. It serves as a communication device for interactions with insurers at the local and national level. The goal of the Consensus Statement is to help ensure that all those who are appropriate candidates for these medications have access to them as early in the disease process as possible.

DISEASE-MODIFYING MEDICATIONS

*   *Immunomodulators* (medications designed to modify the immune system in order to alter the course of MS):

Interferon beta-1a—intramuscular (Avonex®)
Interferon beta-1a—subcutaneous (Rebif®)

Interferon beta-1b (Betaseron®)

Glatiramer acetate (Copaxone®)

- *Immunosuppressant* (medication designed to shut down the immune system temporarily in order to alter the course of MS:

Mitoxantrone (Novantrone®)

RATIONALE

The disease-modifying therapies have demonstrated the following positive outcomes in people with relapsing forms of MS:

- Reduction in the frequency and severity of relapses (also known as attacks or exacerbations).

- Reduction in the numbers of brain lesions as shown on magnetic reonance imaging (MRI).

- Possible reduction in future disability.

Treatment early in the disease course is important because:

- Numerous studies have demonstrated that irreversible damage to nerve axons can occur during early relapses.

- Studies have also shown that lesions can develop and brain atrophy can occur even in those individuals who are not experiencing any symptoms or relapses.

RECOMMENDATIONS

Based on these findings, it is the consensus of researchers and clinicians with expertise in MS that these agents can reduce future disease activity and improve quality of life for many individuals with relapsing forms of MS, including those with secondary progressive disease who continue to have relapses. Therefore, the Executive Committee of the Medical Advisory Board of the National Multiple Sclerosis Society has adopted the following recommendations:

- Treatment should be considered as soon as possible following a definite diagnosis of MS with active disease (i.e., recent relapses and/or new lesions on MRI), and may also be considered for some patients with a first attack who are at high risk of developing MS (known as *clinically isolated syndrome*).

- Insurers should not limit a person's access to medication because of low relapse rate, age, or level of disability.

- Insurers should not require a person to stop a medication while they are determining the person's eligibility for continued coverage of the medication.

- Treatment should be continued unless the person is not benefiting from it, the side effects are intolerable, or a better treatment becomes available.

- All of these Food and Drug Aminstration (FDA)–approved medications should be covered by each insurer so that a physician and patient can determine the most appropriate treatment for that individual.

- Changing from one immunomodulatory therapy to another should occur only for medically appropriate reasons.

- Immunosuppressant therapy with mitoxantrone (Novantrone®) may be considered for some individuals with worsening relapsing MS or with secondary-progressive MS.

- Most individuals with other medical conditions in addition to their MS can safely take these medications.

- None of these medications have been approved by the FDA for use by women who are trying to become pregnant, are pregnant, or are nursing mothers.

THE STATEMENT FROM THE NETWORK OF CANA-DIAN MS CLINICS STAYS THE SAME – IT HAS NOT BEEN UPDATED SINCE 2000.

||||||||||||||||||||||||||||||||||||||||||||||||||||||||||||||||||||||||||||||||||||||||||||||||||||||||||||||||||||

IMMUNOMODULATORS

Interferons Beta   *Interferons* are naturally occurring proteins that are produced when the body reacts to a foreign substance or agent such as a virus. They belong to a class of molecules called *cytokines*, the hormones of the immune system. These cytokines are important regulators of the immune response to viruses and inflammatory conditions. Interferon beta seems to "calm" the immune system, and is referred to as an *immunomodulatory agent.*

Interferon beta-1b
BETASERON®
Betaseron®, a preparation of interferon beta-1b (8 million units, or 250 micrograms [mcg]), was the first medication to be approved for treatment of the MS disease process. Early studies of the drug were carried out on patients with established relapsing-remitting MS. They demonstrated a reduction in the number and severity of attacks, as well as a reduction of the number of lesions seen on the MRI brain scan. Longer term studies are showing some modification in the rate of progression of the disease as well, but these studies are as yet inconclusive. The drug is self-injected under the skin every other day, using a technique similar to the way a person with diabetes uses insulin. It does cause some side effects, which usually are manageable and tolerable. These include mild flu-like symptoms after the injections, which can be relieved by simple analgesics and

lessen with time, and skin reactions at the injection sites, which may persist for days or weeks. The flu-like symptoms almost always disappear with time, but local injection site reactions may continue to occur. About one in four patients will develop antibodies to the drug, and this may necessitate switching to a noninterferon drug such as glatiramer acetate (Copaxone®), as the antibodies decrease the effectiveness of the drug.

Betaseron® has been available only since 1993, so it is still too early to know how beneficial it will be over the longer term, particularly in people who start on the drugs early in the course of the disease.

Interferon beta-1a
AVONEX®

Avonex®, a preparation of interferon beta-1a (6 million units, or 30 mcg), has also been shown to be safe and effective. It is administered weekly by intramuscular injection. Avonex® is approved for the treatment of relapsing-remitting MS to slow the accumulation of physical disability and decrease the frequency of relapses. In a recent study, it was shown to delay a second attack of MS if used soon after a first episode. This first episode is not sufficient to diagnose MS, and is called a clinically isolated syndrome (CIS). People who have had a positive MRI and one episode that looked like an MS attack (CIS) are said to be at risk for having MS. As discussed in Chapter 1, one of the criteria for labeling someone as having clinically definite MS is having had more than one attack. The MRI may sometimes show slight brain shrinkage (brain atrophy) even early in the disease, and early studies suggest that this drug may slow or delay that process. It has the advantage of needing to be injected only once a week. It also has a low risk of antibody formation which may inactivate the effectiveness of the drug. However, some experts believe that higher dosed, more frequently administered drugs may be more effective. It is important to discuss this issue with your physician. The major disadvantage for patients is that Avonex® is

an intramuscular injection (similar to the flu shot), which many find
harder to self-administer than a subcutaneous injection.

REBIF®

Rebif® is similar to natural interferon beta and is administered by
the subcutaneous route three times a week, usually on Monday, Wednes-
day, and Friday. There are two dosage forms available: 6 million units
or 22 mcg and 12 million units or 44 mcg, which are provided ready to
use in a prefilled syringe. The recommended dose is generally 44 mcg
given three times a week in relapsing-remitting MS. This dose demonstrated reduced relapse frequency, slower progression in disability,
and fewer lesions in the brain. The lower dose (22 mcg) given only
once a week has shown some effect in delaying the second attack and
hence the diagnosis of clinically definite MS. Since starting a disease-
modifying therapy at a low dose, and gradually increasing the dose
over time, tends to decrease side effects, a titration pack is available
to facilitate this process. About one in four people may develop antibodies to the drug, which will require consideration of a switch to a
noninterferon medication such as glatiramer acetate (Copaxone®). To
address this issue, a new formulation of Rebif®, which has reduced
development of these antibodies, may be available in 2007. The new
formulation also has reduced injection site reactions.

Glatiramer Acetate   Glatiramer acetate (Copaxone®) is not an
interferon. Rather, it is a *substitute antigen* that mimics myelin basic
protein, an important component of the CNS myelin sheath, a major
immune target in MS. It is given at a dose of 20 mg subcutane-
ously daily by injection under the skin and is well tolerated by most
people. Glatiramer acetate appears to inhibit the CNS immune reactions that are responsible for tissue damage and the production of
MS plaques in people with MS.

It has been shown to reduce both the number of attacks
and the number of brain lesions seen on MRI in patients with
relapsing-remitting MS, but the MRI and clinical parameters take
some time to have effect. Side effects are minimal compared to the

interferons because Copaxone® does not cause the flu-like reactions often seen with those drugs. It can occasionally cause episodes of flushing, palpitations/tachycardia, chest pain, and dyspnea (difficulty breathing), but these are very infrequent and transient and often absent on the next injection.

Natalizumab Natalizumab (Tysabri®) is the newest medicine approved for the treatment of MS. It is an antibody that is thought to inhibit white blood cells from getting into the central nervous system and attacking nerves. Shortly after this promising new agent was released for MS, it was voluntarily withdrawn from the market by the manufacturer as a few patients developed a serious, and often fatal, CNS infection called progressive multifocal leukoencephalopathy (PML). The people who developed PML had a history of taking another drug that would also affect the immune system so the combination was of particular concern. After a careful assessment of all patients on the drug in trials for MS and Crohn's disease did not uncover further cases, it was rereleased first for clinical trails and then for MS treatment, with the caution about additional drugs and for careful monitoring of patients under treatment through a restricted distribution program. The drug has promise because of effectiveness in reducing attacks of MS and improving the MRI profile, but long-term results will await further study It is generally recommended for people who have not been helped by the other MS drugs.

OTHER DISEASE-MODIFYING AGENTS In addition to the four drugs discussed, other agents sometimes are used for more advanced disease. Mitoxantrone and azathioprine are the most common of these. They are discussed here because you may read or hear about them.

Mitoxantrone Mitoxantrone (Novantrone®) is an anticancer drug that also is a strong immune system suppressant. It has been highly effective in suppressing the animal model disease EAE (experimental allergic encephalomyelitis), and encouraging results from several clinical trials showed a marked decrease in active MS lesions on MRI scanning and some reduction in the progression of MS. The drug was approved for use in MS by the FDA in 2000 and generally is reserved for people with MS whose disease is seriously worsening. The long-term use of this drug is limited by the risk of serious cardiac complications, the risk of developing leukemia, and the need to restrict the total dose of the drug over about 2 years. Each infusion of the drug requires prior assessment of the patient's cardiac status.

Azathioprine   Azathioprine (Imuran®) has been available for many decades and has been widely used in Europe but less so in North America. It is not approved for treatment of MS in the United States by the FDA. There is some evidence that it reduces the number of attacks of MS and may reduce disability from the disease to some extent. The effect is modest at best, and in trials it took years to see benefits over those not receiving the therapy. It comes in pill form, is easy to use, and is inexpensive. However, there has been concern that this immunosuppressant might increase the incidence of certain malignancies (such as lymphomas) if it is taken on a long-term basis. Recent European studies have not shown such an increase, so its use is increasing. Regular blood tests are required when a patient is receiving this medication to detect early indications of liver dysfunction or effects on the blood counts. There are trials underway to assess the effect of combining azathioprine with an interferon.

Management of Symptoms

The most common symptoms of MS include numbness, fatigue, weakness, blurred vision, poor balance, bladder frequency and urgency, and difficulty walking. It is important to recognize that although a wide range of symptoms may occur with MS, a given individual may experience only some of them and never have others. Some symptoms may occur once, resolve, and never return. Because it is such an individual disease, it is not helpful—and may be misleading and frightening—to compare yourself with someone else, who often will have different symptoms, a different pattern of disease activity, and a different pattern of progression.

MOBILITY

Weakness It is common for a person with MS to have symptoms of weakness in one or both legs. Initially this may be transient, lasting days or weeks during an attack, but in some people, weakness progresses over many years as a major symptom. Because the nerves in the CNS have important function in the motor control over muscles, patches of demyelination may affect these fibers and cause weakness in different muscle groups, most commonly in the legs. In some people, especially those who develop the disease after the age of 40, leg weakness and spasticity may be the only symptoms of MS, progressing slowly without any acute attacks.

It is common to develop weakness during an attack of MS, but sometimes weakness may be present all the time. The pattern of weakness can be asymmetrical, involving one limb or one side more than the other, or it can seem to be only in the legs. If it comes on in an acute attack, it is treated with IV steroids. If it is persistent, it is important for the neurologist to decide how much is related to weakness in the muscles, how much is due to spasticity or increased tone in the muscles, and how much is contributed by a change in sensation that makes the limbs seem more clumsy.

If weakness is present, you should be encouraged to increase your level of exercise to strengthen the muscles. A physical therapist can help if you experience a lot of weakness, but if the weakness is mild, you can do an exercise program on your own. It is important to remember that any muscle can be strengthened. Just as "normal" muscles can be made stronger by exercise, weak ones also can be trained and strengthened by exercise. The muscles may not return to normal, but they will be stronger than they otherwise would have been, and that is always worthwhile.

If there is a lot of weakness in a limb, various aids, such as an ankle brace for footdrop or a cane, may be necessary to help with walking until improvement is seen. Footdrop usually is first noticed when "tripping" over your foot occurs, causing the tips of shoes on the affected side to become scraped or scuffed. If weakness persists after treatment with steroids, a referral for physical therapy may be arranged so that the problems can be assessed, an exercise program developed, and any immediate problems treated.

You should continue a regular exercise program even after weakness has improved (see A Note About Exercise later in this chapter).

Spasticity   A complex control of muscle movements normally allows some muscles to contract and others to relax when a movement is carried out. This normal pattern can be disrupted when nerves in the CNS are damaged by MS, resulting in the simultaneous contraction of many muscles, both the ones that help (agonists) and those that oppose the movement (antagonists). This causes the "tone" to increase in all the muscles, the limb to feel tight, and the limb movements to be slower and less smooth. It is more difficult and more tiring to walk with legs that have spasticity.

Spasticity can be reduced by exercise and by normal use of the muscles. It is important to perform stretching exercises of the spastic, tight muscles to prevent *contractures*, a state in which the tight muscle shortens. Each muscle should be stretched fully and held for a minute (See A Note About Exercise later in this chapter).

A number of medications that are considered muscle relaxants do not work well in MS and can have side effects. An effective medication for spasticity and the symptoms that it produces (spasms, cramps, pain, aching) is baclofen, which can be taken in different ways depending on the symptoms, their severity, and the person's tolerance to the medication. Because some people have painful spasms only at night and minor spasticity in the daytime, a nightly dose may be all that is needed. Others need relief from spasticity all the time, and a schedule of multiple doses a day is developed. Because all patients can reach a dosage level that seems too high, causing a general feeling of weakness and drowsiness, your doctor may start you with a very low dose, perhaps half a tablet (5 mg) twice a day, and slowly increase by adding a further half tablet every 3 or 4 days until symptoms are reasonably controlled. If symptoms are helped at a low dose, the dose will be held there. If you develop side effects when the dose is increased, they may be eliminated by skipping a dose and going back to the previous level. Baclofen is very helpful in reducing the spasms and pain sometimes associated with spasticity, but it is only somewhat helpful in improving function that has been limited by spasticity.

Tizanidine (Zanaflex®) up is also an effective antispasticity agent that has effects similar to those of baclofen. It is especially effective for night spasms and sometimes is effective in reducing spasticity in patients who do not respond to other agents. Its use in combination with low doses of baclofen may produce an optimal antispasticity effect with fewer side effects. Tizanidine may cause a feeling of tiredness, which can be minimized by slowly increasing the dose as this therapy begins.

Disturbances of Balance and Gait Disturbances of gait and balance are common in MS because they can be caused by changes in different parts of the nervous system. A person may notice that he or she does not walk or stand as steadily if experiencing incoordination, weakness in one or more limbs, numbness, dizziness, vertigo, or even visual problems. One of the most troublesome causes of gait disturbance is spasticity in the muscles of the legs. For some people, this is the most limiting problem of MS. Because so much of what we do involves being mobile, this problem causes the most disability and handicap in the disease over the lifetime of many (but not all) people with MS.

In many instances, difficulty in walking comes with the various symptoms of an attack of MS, improving or clearing as the attack settles down. In other instances, it is an ongoing problem. A person with MS may have few other problems except a gait difficulty that slowly increases over a period of years. This pattern is more common in those who develop the disease later in life.

Physical therapy can be helpful for gait difficulty, and a physical therapist can show you techniques of gait training, muscle strengthening, exercises, safety hints, and the use of mobility aids.

A Note About Exercise   Exercise is important for everyone, especially a person with MS. A program of range-of-motion exercises is one exercise program that you should do daily, or even more than once a day if your muscles are very stiff. Each joint is put through its full range-of- motion to keep it healthy and lubricated and to stretch and loosen the muscles that move the joints.

A simple exercise program that anyone can manage is the 10-10-20 exercise program, in which 10 general exercises are performed, each for 10 repetitions, for a duration of a 20-minute exercise period. The 10 exercises are general ones that improve overall fitness. They can be altered according to individual capacity and the need to overcome specific problems or weak areas. They can be individually designed by a physical therapist and modified as needed.

Swimming has a number of advantages, although it often is more difficult to arrange on a regular basis. Swimming exercises most muscles, and some movements and exercises can be done more easily in water because the water supports the body during movement. The water should be cool because most people with MS are sensitive to heat and may be bothered by exercises that increase body heat or by warm exercise rooms. Function may be improved just by cooling in a swimming pool. Although swimming in the ocean can have the same effect, waves can easily put you off balance.

Relaxation techniques are useful and improve the enjoyment and rewards of a regular exercise program. They involve methods of learning positive relaxation of the mind and body, deep breathing, and mental imagery, combined with alternating contraction and relaxation of various muscles.

An exercise program should be regular and enjoyable. Anyone can carry out a boring exercise program for a few weeks, but not for a lifetime—which is what we all need to do. That is why many basements have a corner with almost new exercise equipment gathering dust. Some machines look terrific, but they are not very enjoyable to use, and sometimes we think that it is the machines (or physiotherapists) that are going to make us strong. YOU do the exercises, not the machine.

Exercise programs that many people enjoy include swimming, mat exercises, walking, and tai chi, but you must think about the exercises that you would find most enjoyable and can imagine still doing regularly years from now.

SENSORY SYMPTOMS

Numbness　The term *numbness* covers many alterations to the sensory system that affect sensation, particularly in the skin. People may experience numbness, but more often they feel tingling, pins and needles, burning, coldness, or other sensations that are difficult to describe. The disruption to the sensory nerves can be caused by damage to the spinal cord, the brain stem, or the brain itself.

Tingling and numbness are "normal" symptoms that virtually everyone has experienced (a leg falling "asleep," dental anesthesia, cold feet in the winter), but these common occurrences are due to pressure, anesthetics, or cold to a peripheral nerve in an arm or leg, whereas MS affects the myelin of the nerves (and sometimes the underlying nerves) in the CNS. It may seem as if the nerve in the leg (the peripheral nervous system) is affected in MS, but in fact the demyelination is in the CNS. Numbness most often is felt in the ends of the limbs, the feet and lower legs, or the hands, but it can seem to rise from the legs up to the upper abdomen. Sometimes the numbness seems to have a level, as if a belt of numbness were wrapped around the abdomen; it also may be painful, with decreased sensation below the level.

Although numbness often is only a brief annoyance, it can cause other problems if it persists or only partially clears. You may drop things when your hands and fingertips are numb, even light objects such as paper, because you do not know how tightly you are gripping them. Because feeling in your fingers is decreased, you may need to use your vision to help recognize things that you could identify previously with your fingertips. You may have trouble identifying objects in your purse or pocket because numbness can decrease your ability to recognize a comb or a coin by its characteristic feel. You may not realize that good balance involves sensing information about the muscles and tendons in the limbs, which is carried to the nervous system by sensory nerves. If numbness is present in the legs, people use their eyes to maintain good balance, and tend to look down as they walk. On the other hand, they will have more difficulty if they look up or around, and if they walk on uneven ground or in the dark.

Numbness occasionally is accompanied by disagreeable sensations called *dysesthesias*, such as burning, "creepy-crawly" feelings, or sensitive skin (sensations similar to those felt when dental anesthesia is wearing off). These disagreeable feelings usually improve as sensation improves, but they sometimes require treatment. When numbness or dysesthesias occur as part of an acute attack, it usually improves with intravenous (IV) steroids. More persistent disagreeable sensations may be reduced by a tricyclic antidepressant such as amytriptyline (Elavil®). This medication, although an antidepressant, has other beneficial effects and is useful in pain syndromes and migraine as well as disturbing sensory problems.

Some changes in sensation are described as pain, which is discussed later in this chapter. One of these is the symptom of an electric shock–like feeling in the back or limbs on flexing the neck.

This occurs when there is some inflammation in the posterior columns of the cervical spinal cord, and the bending of the neck stretches these inflamed fibers, causing them to fire. The symptom is called *Lhermitte's phenomenon,* after the French neurologist who described it. It often is transient, clearing when the inflammation abates, and can be made to clear faster with IV steroids.

Facial Numbness A common and upsetting symptom in MS is numbness on one side of the face. However, this is a minor symptom that usually clears without treatment. You might have a tingling feeling or a numbness, often described as similar to dental anesthesia, which at times can involve the gums and tongue. Symptoms around the face are perceived as more disturbing to people than the same degree of numbness elsewhere, such as the foot or hand, but facial numbness often goes away in days or a few weeks. The neurologist may also find subtle differences to various sensations in the face on examination, of which the person is unaware.

Vision Loss Several types of vision problems may occur in MS. *Optic neuritis* (sometimes called retrobulbar neuritis) is an episode of demyelination in the optic nerve behind the eyeball. Because it occurs in the nerve, a physician looking in the eye during the first episode may not see anything wrong. Later, some scarring may occur in the optic nerve, and it will look pale in the back of the eye, when seen by the doctor through a hand-held instrument called an ophthalmoscope. High-dose IV steroids is the standard treatment when one eye or occasionally both eyes are affected. Symptoms include blurred vision, loss of peripheral or "side" vision, and one or more black or "blind" spots. Total loss of vision in one eye may occur in some instances, but this will usually improve with time. Optic neuritis sometimes also causes pain in the eye, which clears quickly when steroid treatment is begun. Vision returns more slowly. It is common for individuals with relapsing-remitting MS to have one or more episodes of optic neuritis, although many people never experience this problem.

Another visual complaint people with MS may experience is a vague feeling that their vision is not as clear as it should be, even if a recent eye examination indicates vision to be normal. The problem may be with certain contrasts in the visual fields, or with color, which causes a mild change that usually is not detected on standard eye tests. When this occurs, text with sharp contrast is easiest to read. A related symptom is a decrease in vision associated with exercise (Uhthoff's phenomenon), which is probably related to an increase in body heat,that affects nerve conduction. Vision returns when the person stops exercising and cools down.

Some people with MS experience double vision and complain that they cannot see well. Actually, the vision in each eye separately may be normal, but the eyes do not focus together. Although it is annoying, double vision usually clears on its own or responds to IV steroids. It is rarely a persistent problem and can be temporarily relieved by patching one eye.

Another problem with eye control that may be experienced as a visual problem is *nystagmus*. When your physician asks you to move your eyes in different directions, he or she is testing eye movements and control. Nystagmus is a regular fine jerkiness of the eyes that may occur when looking to the sides, which usually is not noticed by the patient. Sometimes the eyes operate differently in that situation, with one having more jerkiness than the other. This causes a sensation that the environment is moving (oscillopsia) or looks double when looking to the sides. In some people, the pupillary response to light is slowed, experienced as difficulty with bright lights, especially while driving at night. Glasses with photosensitive lenses usually compensate for this problem.

All that affects vision is not MS, and you should have regular eye examinations to see if you need glasses to correct the vision changes and eye problems that occur in all of us with age.

Pain   At one time, it was believed that pain was unusual in MS. We now know that pain, in one form or another, occurs in more than half of all people who have the disease. It may take the form of an aching in muscles, shooting pains, jabbing facial pain, or discomfort from burning, tingling, or other sensory changes. The first step is to determine the specific cause of the pain. Not all pain is the result of MS, so other problems must be considered. Since pain problems in MS have specific treatments, as does pain from other causes, it is important to identify the underlying cause.

The spasms and cramps in the large muscles of the legs that occur when tone is increased by spasticity can be reduced by physical therapy, exercise, relaxation techniques, passive stretching, massage, and local cold. The pain associated with spasticity can often be effectively reduced with baclofen or tizanidine (Zanaflex®).

Remember that not all symptoms in people with MS are due to the disease and that any problems that cause pain in anyone else also can occur. Joint pain, back pain, abdominal pain, headaches, and other problems may be due to conditions that have nothing to do with MS and should be investigated and treated just as they would if MS were not present.

Facial Pain   A type of nerve pain that can occur in the face, called *trigeminal neuralgia,* is characterized by a sharp, jabbing, knife-like pain, usually over the cheek and sometimes over the eye on one side. Although it can occur as an isolated syndrome in the elderly, it often indicates the underlying demyelinating process of MS in a younger person. Several types of pain occur in the face, including temporomandibular joint (TMJ) pain, tension headache, and migraine. If trigeminal neuralgia is the cause, it is treated with a group of medications that decrease the nerve firing. The initial treatment usually is carbamazepine (Tegretol®), to which most people quickly respond well. In those few people who have unacceptable side effects, baclofen, diphenylhydantoin (Dilantin®), gabapentin (Neurontin®), or duloxetine hydrochloride (Cimbalta®) is substituted.

A small number of people do not tolerate these medications, lose the beneficial drug effect over time, or do not respond to them.

In such cases, a surgical procedure may be considered. It usually is done on an outpatient basis by a needle procedure through the face into the trigeminal (fifth cranial) nerve. This is usually successful. Trigeminal neuralgia associated with MS is due to the presence of a plaque in the connections of the fifth cranial nerve in the brain stem. Although it can cause severe facial pain, trigeminal neuralgia usually is successfully managed. It is not uncommon for the problem to return months or years after it has been controlled, but treatment can be restarted if it does.

Hearing Changes   It is unusual for people with MS to notice any change in hearing other than that seen in the normal population, but MS can on occasion cause a decrease in hearing. More commonly, a subtle change can be noted on specific testing of the hearing system, but without producing noticeable symptoms. Significant hearing change due to MS is rarely a problem and, when acute episodes of hearing loss do occur, full recovery can be expected.

BLADDER AND BOWEL ISSUES

Bladder Control   The most common symptoms of bladder involvement in MS are the need to urinate *often* (frequency) and the need to urinate *now* (urgency). If these symptoms are particularly troublesome, involuntary wetting (incontinence) can occur because of difficulty getting to the bathroom in time. Many people manage this by being aware of their symptoms and taking opportunities to urinate regularly. Markedly restricting fluid intake, which seems to be a logical method of dealing with the problem, is actually a bad idea; your kidneys and bladder need a continuous flow of fluids to excrete wastes and minimize the opportunity for infection.

If frequency and urgency are more serious problems than you can manage by simple measures, medications such as oxybutynin chloride (Ditropan®), propantheline bromide (Probanthine®), tolterodine tartrate (Detrol®), or flavoxate hydrochloride (Urispas®) may control the problem. It is important to determine that urinary retention is not present before these medications are initiated. A number of problems with the bladder can occur in MS, each of which needs a specific approach to management. If simple measures and these medications are not sufficient to control the problem, a urologic assessment is needed to see if other approaches are required.

It is important to know that bladder problems are common in MS and that they can be managed with simple measures in most cases, but also that they can lead to serious complications if untreated. Urinary infection in men should always be explored further, and recurrent urinary tract infection in women also requires investigation. If burning or painful urination occurs, especially when the urine is cloudy and has a foul odor, you probably have a bladder infection and need to be in touch with your physician right away.

Bladder symptoms sometimes can be reduced by drinking about eight glasses (8 oz) of fluid daily, limiting citrus juices (orange, grapefruit, and tomato juices), and adding cranberry juice or cranberry tablets several times daily.

Bowel Control   Bowel control problems (primarily constipation) are less common than bladder problems, and in most cases they also can be managed by simple methods. The first step is to maintain a regular bowel schedule. Try to have a bowel movement each day after breakfast because establishing a regular daily pattern avoids constipation and a tendency to irregular bowel movements as a result of inactivity. Each day take the time to sit and try at the same time—do not wait until you feel like going to the bathroom—try to develop a regular reflex timing for bowel movements. Your diet should be high in fiber, including a serving of bran each day, and there should be adequate fruits and vegetables in your meals. Drinking enough fluids is also critical, as dry stool is the most common cause of constipation.

Another factor in bowel health is exercise—this helps maintain good bowel function in everyone, but it is especially important when you have MS. Loss of bowel control is a more serious problem and can be managed by altering diet and some exercises, and in some cases medication will help. A consultation with a gastroenterologist may be needed because this problem can discourage a person from taking part in many social and family activities.

OTHER SYMPTOMS

Fatigue People with MS may notice two patterns of fatigue. One is a feeling of tiredness and weakness that occurs with increasing exercise or other physical activity. For instance, walking may be fine at the onset, but your legs may become increasingly heavy and tired after walking a long distance, with some dragging of the feet. Strength is recovered and you can continue again after sitting down and resting for a brief time.

Another kind of fatigue is a general feeling of exhaustion, which can be more annoying and limiting. This can be mild or severe, intermittent or continuous. You may experience this type of fatigue quite suddenly during a normal day, which may come over you like a wave, making it difficult to continue with whatever you are doing. More commonly, a general fatigue is present no matter how much or how little you do. It may be aggravated by overdoing activity or getting less sleep, but it may be present even if you do nothing and have had a good night's sleep. When we ask people with MS to list the symptoms that bother them the most, fatigue usually is at the top of the list; it also is the most common.

Most people learn to modify their day in ways that allow them to manage fatigue, such as taking brief rests or even occasional naps. Others say that they cannot do this because of the nature of their work or responsibilities, and they push through the fatigue without its causing any problems. It simply makes you tired to overdo it when you have fatigue; it does not worsen your MS. The most common problem from overdoing things is to be more tired. It is common for people to say they can push through their work or task but that they pay for this effort with several days of increased fatigue. Sometimes the fatigue will characteristically appear at about the same time of day, allowing for some restructuring of activities if your work or other schedules permit.

Most people with MS say that the fatigue they experience feels abnormal, unlike the normal tiredness that everyone experiences. Most neurologic diseases are not associated with this pattern of tiredness, although a number of other autoimmune diseases do exhibit this unusual fatigue. Because it is so "different" and so common in MS, it is surprising that it was not recognized as a characteristic symptom of MS until recently. By a serendipitous observation, it was found that amantadine (formerly sold as Symmetrel®) taken twice a day is helpful in reducing fatigue in about half the people who experience it. Another medication that may be helpful is modafinil (Provigil®), a drug originally developed for narcolepsy. It has not been available long enough to assess its long-term value. There is some suggestion that high doses of enteric-coated aspirin (ECASA) (Entrophen®) may be helpful, but caution must be used with long-term high doses.

Cognitive Impairment People with MS, sometimes even those with a new diagnosis, may experience difficulty remembering things, finding the right words, or concentrating. These problems might reflect *cognitive impairment*—problems with thinking and memory that occur in about 50 to 60 percent of people with MS, which are generally unrelated to disease duration or seriousness of other symptoms. Fortunately, most people do not have extensive difficulty, and compensatory activities can be introduced, such as establishing regular routines (e.g., always putting the house keys in the same place), relying more on written information (such as written driving directions), and using a day calendar to track important activities. Formal testing can be done to identify any problems you are having so that a management plan can be tailored to your needs. If you are concerned about cognitive function, discuss this with your MS doctor, nurse, or mental health professional so that the issue can be addressed. (see *Multiple Sclerosis: Understanding Cognitive Challenges* in Additional Readings).

Tremor   Everyone has some tremor (to see the normal physiologic tremor, put a piece of paper on top of your outstretched hand). Multiple sclerosis may be accompanied by different types of tremor, ranging from annoying to fairly disabling. There are a variety of approaches to controlling them, some of which people learn on their own. For example, bracing the forearm against the side or on a hard surface reduces arm and hand tremor. Another variation is to have a method of immobilization that is used for some specific task, such as writing, but is removed when the task is completed. Physical and occupational therapists may use *patterning*, repeating movements to make them smoother and more automatic. Adding weights to the limb may reduce tremor, and adaptive equipment can be useful.

Medication is only partially effective, and some of the drugs tried in the past seemed to give only limited assistance and caused side effects. Perhaps the only drugs that may have a significant effect are beta blockers such as propranolol (Inderal®). Mild sedatives and tranquilizers may help, but they probably are only worthwhile when you have some other need for a sedative, such as tension or anxiety, that aggravate tremor. Stereotactic brain surgery has been used in selected cases, but this is unusual and carries significant risk.

Vertigo   Vertigo is the sensation that many people call "dizziness," but since that term can mean different things, it is necessary to explain exactly what you feel. Vertigo has the sensation of movement, whether it seems that the room is moving or turning or that *you* seem to be moving. If it is severe, the room seems to be spinning, or you may feel like you are tipping or falling or that the floor is coming up to meet you. This sensation usually is due to a disturbance in the vestibular system of the middle ear or its connections within the brain stem and brain. In MS, the problem most often is in the nerve connections in the brain stem. It usually is transient, lasting hours or occasionally weeks; it is unusual for it to last much longer. If it persists, it can be treated by stimulating the vestibular system or by suppressing the vestibular reflexes with medication.

If the onset of vertigo is acute and lasts for many days, it can be treated by intravenous (IV) steroids, but it usually resolves by itself. When vertigo is worsened by movement, as it often is, paradoxically the problem can be reduced by purposely stimulating the vertigo. Thus, positional exercises can be done using a simple method on a soft surface such as a bed. The vestibular system is stimulated by falling onto the bed to one side three times (the vertigo lessens each time), then to the other side, and then backward. There often is a position of comfort when a person has vertigo, with fewer symptoms when lying on one side and more symptoms when lying on the other side, and with the head supported at a certain angle. Sedatives are helpful, as is diazepam (Valium®), which suppresses the vestibular reflex.

Vertigo can be mild, experienced as a slight swimming feeling in the head. Mild nausea and poor concentration often are associated with this. Again, positional exercises and an exercise program are more helpful than sitting still, which is the natural tendency.

Seizures   Seizures are not common in MS; they occur in only approximately 6 percent of patients. They usually are effectively treated with common anticonvulsants such as phenytoin (Dilantin®) or carbamazepine (Tegretol®). An unusual type of "seizure" is a localized spasm that is more like a major muscle spasm than an epileptic seizure and often occurs on one side of the body. Such spasms also respond to medication such as carbamazepine.

Facial Weakness   Facial weakness can occur suddenly in MS, although it is uncommon. When it does happen, especially early in the course of the disease, it may resemble Bell's palsy, a benign form of acute facial palsy that often follows a viral infection. Both Bell's palsy and the facial weakness of MS respond to steroids. In MS, no treatment may be needed if the weakness is mild or is already rapidly improving on its own.

Summary

MS brings with it many uncertainties about the future. However, what is certain is that MS is a treatable disease, with many new therapies on the horizon. You have every reason to be optimistic about your future, in that currently available medications have already helped thousands of people with their MS, and to actively seek help for all ramifications of the disease. Be sure you have the best health-care team for your needs, then work closely with them, and your MS Society, to maintain the highest possible quality of life.

4

||||||||||||||||||||||||||||||||||||||||||||||||||||||||||||||||||||||||||||||||||||||||||||||||||||||||||||||||

Unconventional Therapies and Multiple Sclerosis

P eople who are recently diagnosed with multiple sclerosis (MS) often leave no stone unturned in their search for effective treatments for their disease. One area of exploration for you may be unconventional therapies. Among these therapies, there is much variability in the quality of available information and also in its effectiveness, safety, and cost. Consequently, it is especially important to be knowledgeable and cautious in this area. This chapter provides background information about unconventional medicine, strategies for evaluating unconventional therapies, and MS-specific information about unconventional therapies that are popular or are particularly relevant to MS.

Definition of Unconventional Medicine

Unconventional medicine is a term that is surprisingly difficult to define. Part of the difficulty is that many different terms are used in this area. In addition to *unconventional medicine*, other frequently used terms include *alternative medicine, complementary medicine*, and *integrative medicine.*

One of the more commonly used terms is *unconventional medicine.* This is sometimes defined as therapies that are not typically taught in medical schools or generally available in hospitals. However, this definition is awkward because it states what unconventional medicine *is not* as opposed to what it *is*. Also, this definition is a "moving target" because it depends on the medical traditions of the country in which it is used, and in some countries, including the United States, many medical schools now offer courses in unconventional medicine.

There are many other definitions of unconventional medicine. One definition that is more precise, but also more complex, is provided by the National Institutes of Health (NIH). In this definition, unconventional medicine is subdivided into categories. These categories, with representative examples, include:

- Biologically based therapies: dietary supplements, diets, bee venom therapy

- Mind-body therapies: guided imagery, hypnosis, meditation

- Alternative medical systems: traditional Chinese medicine, ayurveda, homeopathy

- Manipulative and body-based therapies: chiropractic, reflexology, massage

- Energy therapies: therapeutic touch, magnets

Other terms refer to the way in which the therapies are used. Unconventional therapies that are used instead of conventional medicine are known as *alternative medicine*, while unconventional therapies that are used in conjunction with conventional medicine are called *complementary medicine*. A broader term is *complementary and alternative medicine* (CAM). An even broader term, *integrative medicine*, refers to the combined use of conventional and unconventional medicine.

There have been many studies of the use of CAM in the general population and in people with MS. In studies in several countries, it has been found that about one-half to three-fourths of people with MS use some form of unconventional medicine. Nearly all people with MS use unconventional medicine in conjunction with conventional medicine. In other words, the unconventional medicine is used as *complementary medicine.*

Evidence for the Safety and Effectiveness of Therapies

Different types of evidence may be available to determine the safety and effectiveness of unconventional as well as conventional therapies. When considering a therapy, it is extremely important to understand these different levels of evidence and how they apply specifically to MS. Information about a therapy may be based on theoretical arguments, experimental studies, or clinical trials of people with MS.

When reviewing information about a therapy, it is important to determine the strength of available evidence. Some CAM literature does not distinguish between the various levels of evidence or makes very strong recommendations on the basis of weak evidence. For example, a CAM therapy such as a dietary supplement might be highly recommended for MS because it suppresses the immune system, produces therapeutic effects in the animal model of MS, and has minimal side effects. Although this sounds promising, there is no clinical trial evidence. As a result, it is quite likely that this therapy would *not* be recommended for MS.

Ideally, there should be high-quality clinical evidence for well-tolerated therapies that could cure MS and completely eliminate all MS symptoms. Unfortunately, this is not the case. Therefore, there are circumstances in which conventional medicine uses approaches that are not entirely proven. These approaches must be used thoughtfully and with recognition of the limited evidence, with careful weighing of possible risks and benefits. The most common example of these unproven conventional approaches is the use of symptomatic therapies for which there is limited clinical evidence ("off-label" use).

People with MS who are interested in CAM should use a careful and thoughtful approach that is similar to that used for conventional therapies for which the evidence is limited. It is important to obtain unbiased MS-relevant information, evaluate the safety and effectiveness of the therapy, and discuss the therapy with your physician or other conventional health-care provider. If a therapy is pursued, there should be a plan for monitoring for a response. If that response does not occur, the therapy should be discontinued and other approaches should be considered. It is important to use caution, realize that the safety and effectiveness information about most CAM therapies is limited, and recognize that there is a certain degree of risk in pursuing CAM therapy.

Using Complementary and Alternative Medicine

It is important to know when it may be reasonable to use CAM; for example, for symptoms such as mild fatigue or mild muscle stiffness, or for conditions for which conventional medicine has no effective therapies or only partially effective therapies. On the other hand, a serious disease such as MS should not be treated initially or exclusively with CAM therapies.

Some CAM books make erroneous claims about MS, some of which are potentially dangerous. One frequent misunderstanding is that MS, as an immune disease, should be treated by stimulating the immune system with dietary supplements. *This is incorrect.* MS is an immune disease, but it is characterized by *excessive* immune system activity. As a result, effective MS therapies generally *decrease* immune system activity.

Features of some CAM therapies that should raise concerns:

- "Secret ingredients" or little objective information about safety or effectiveness

- Extremely strong claims about effectiveness, such as claims that a single therapy is effective for many different conditions

- Use of "testimonials" in which individuals make strong claims about effectiveness

- Much cost or effort is involved, such as inpatient therapy or intravenous treatment

There are common misconceptions about dietary supplements, which include vitamins, minerals, and herbs. Some supplements are claimed to have therapeutic effects and no side effects, which is not true. Supplements, especially herbs, are similar to medications and contain chemicals that may produce beneficial effects but may also cause side effects. Also, it is sometimes claimed that "more is better," especially with vitamins and minerals. This is not correct and may actually be dangerous. High doses of many supplements may produce side effects. Finally, it is sometimes stated that natural compounds are safe and beneficial. In fact, there are many products that are natural but are also very toxic. Examples include mercury, arsenic, animal venoms, and poisonous mushrooms.

Unconventional Therapies Relevant to MS

For some individuals, the thoughtful use of CAM therapies, especially in combination with conventional medicine, may allow for an individualized treatment plan and provide hope, control, and a sense of empowerment. The remainder of this chapter will provide MS-relevant information about CAM therapies that have been specifically studied in MS, are used commonly in the general population or by people with MS, or raise specific safety concerns.

Acupuncture and Traditional Chinese Medicine

Acupuncture is one component of traditional Chinese medicine (TCM). Other components include traditional Chinese herbs, nutrition, exercise, stress reduction, and massage. TCM is based on a theory of body function that is very different from that of Western medicine. Specifically, it is believed that energy, or *qi*, flows through 14 major pathways, or *meridians*, on the body. There is also a balance of opposites, which are known as *yin* and *yang*. According to TCM, disease occurs when there is disturbance or disharmony of energy. With acupuncture, thin, metallic needles are inserted in specific points on the meridians. It is believed that the insertion of acupuncture needles alters the flow of energy in such a way that it produces therapeutic effects.

There is limited information about acupuncture in people with MS. Two recent preliminary studies indicate that 20 to 25 percent of people with MS have tried acupuncture. Two older studies reported beneficial effects of acupuncture in people with MS, but these findings are not definitive because the studies were small and not rigorously designed. A more recent preliminary study suggests that acupuncture may improve the symptoms of MS-related bladder dysfunction. In people who do not have MS, several studies indicate that acupuncture improves pain, nausea, and vomiting. Studies of Chinese herbal medicine in MS are also limited. Some studies, published in Chinese, report that Chinese herbal therapy decreases the attack rate and slows the progression of the disease. These studies are difficult to evaluate because they are not available in English.

Acupuncture is usually well tolerated, especially when it is done by a well-trained acupuncturist. Sterile needles should be used to avoid infections, including hepatitis and AIDS. Acupuncture is moderately expensive. The safety of Chinese herbal medicine has not been well characterized, especially in people with MS. There is a theoretical risk of worsening MS with immune-stimulating herbs, which include Asian ginseng, astragalus, and maitake and reishi mushrooms. In addition, one herb that mildly suppresses the immune system, thunder god vine, *Tripterygium wilfordii*, may produce serious side effects, including death. Chinese herbal medicine is a low-cost therapy.

Marijuana (Cannabis)

For years, it has been claimed that marijuana, also known as *cannabis*, is an effective treatment for MS. Marijuana, which is illegal in many countries, contains compounds known as cannabinoids. These compounds, which include tetrahydrocannabinol (THC), produce specific biochemical effects in the body. Marijuana may be smoked or ingested. There are prescription medications that contain cannabinoids. In the United States, THC is available as dronabinol (Marinol®). In Europe, Canada, and Australia, a synthetic form of THC is available as nabilone (Cesamet®). An oral spray form of cannabis, Sativex®, has been approved for use in Canada for treating MS pain.

Cannabinoids exert several biologicl effects that, on a theoretical basis, could be therapeutic for MS. First, they bind to proteins in the central nervous system that suppress excessive nerve cell activity. This could, on a theoretical basis, decrease some MS symptoms such as pain and muscle stiffness (spasticity). Also, cannabinoids bind to another type of protein on immune cells and mildly suppress the immune system. It is possible that cannabinoids are able to slow down the disease process in MS through this mechanism. Finally, cannabinoids may protect against nerve cell injury by decreasing the damage caused by an injurious form of nerve cell activity.

There are mixed results in studies of the actual disease in humans. In several surveys of people with MS who have smoked marijuana, symptoms commonly reported to be improved include pain, spasticity, depression, and anxiety. Importantly, surveys such as this are not rigorous enough to provide definitive evidence for effectiveness. Actual clinical studies of the effects of smoked or oral marijuana on MS symptoms are of variable quality. Some, but not all, of these studies have found improvement in spasticity.

Significant risks are associated with smoking marijuana, including nausea, vomiting, sedation, increased risk of seizures, and poor pregnancy outcomes. Driving may be impaired for up to 8 hours after smoking marijuana. High doses of marijuana may impair heart function, decrease reaction time, and produce coordination and visual difficulties. Chronic marijuana use may cause heart attacks, impair lung function, cause dependence and apathy, and increase the risk of cancer of the lung, head, and neck. Smoked marijuana and prescription medications containing cannabinoids are of low-moderate cost.

Chiropractic Medicine

Chiropractic medicine is one of the most popular forms of CAM in the United States. Chiropractic medicine is based on the concept that the nervous system plays a critical role in health and that many diseases are caused by abnormal pressure of bones on the nerves in the spine.

Chiropractors believe that misalignments of the bones of the spine cause abnormal pressure on the nerves that travel from the spinal cord to the muscles and organs of the body which results in impaired muscle and organ function. Spinal manipulation techniques, known as "adjustments," are thought to normalize bone positions and restore normal function.

There are no well-designed studies that document that spinal manipulation or other chiropractic methods can alter the disease course in MS. Isolated clinical reports have described improvement in some MS symptoms with chiropractic treatment, but there are no systematic clinical studies of chiropractic treatment for MS symptoms.

Chiropractic treatment is generally well tolerated. Between 1900 and 1980, 135 complications associated with chiropractic therapy were reported in the medical literature. One of the more common adverse effects is achy muscles, which may be present for 1 to 2 days after manipulation. A rare, but serious, complication associated with neck manipulation is stroke. Very rarely, low back manipulation may cause compression of the nerves of the lower spine (cauda equine syndrome). Pregnant women, people taking anticoagulant medications, and people with spinal bone fractures, spine trauma, significant disc herniations, bone cancer or infection, severe osteoporosis, and severe arthritis should avoid chiropractic therapy. Importantly, since chiropractors are not as well trained in diagnosis as physicians, people with serious diseases or conditions should be evaluated and treated by a physician and should not substitute chiropractic medicine for conventional medicine. Chiropractic therapy is of low-moderate cost.

Cooling Therapy

Cooling therapy is a form of CAM that is unique to MS. It has been known for years that changes in body temperature may significantly affect MS symptoms. Specifically, small increases in body temperature ($32.9°F$, $0.5°C$) may worsen symptoms, while small decreases may improve symptoms. Consequently, various cooling methods have been developed. These methods range from simple techniques, such as drinking cold liquids and staying in air-conditioned areas, to complex methods, such as using specially designed cooling suits. Cooling suits may be *passive* or *active*. Passive garments use evaporation or ice packs for cooling; active garments use circulating coolants.

Beneficial effects of cooling garments have been noted in several clinical studies. Unfortunately, some of these reports are preliminary and most of the studies have been small and not rigorously conducted. Among these studies, improvement in fatigue is frequently seen. Other symptoms showing improvement include leg weakness, spasticity, difficulty walking, bladder dysfunction, sexual difficulties, visual changes, speech difficulties, cognitive difficulties, and incoordination. The results of the most rigorous cooling study in MS have been recently published. In this study, on the basis of objective measures, cooling was associated with mildly improved walking and visual function. By subjective measures, cooling improved fatigue, strength, and cognition. Cooling garments may be especially well suited for those who are heat sensitive.

The use of cooling garments is usually well tolerated. Some people feel uncomfortable when cooling begins, and handling of the garments may be cumbersome. Some people with MS have a paradoxical sensitivity to cold, in which case cooling may actually *worsen* symptoms. Costs of cooling are dependent on the method used. Simple techniques are of low cost. Cooling garments are of moderate cost. Passive garments are generally less expensive than active garments.

Dental Amalgam Removal

Removal of dental amalgam has been proposed as a treatment method for MS. For more than 150 years, cavities have been filled with dental amalgam, which is composed of mercury as well as silver, copper, tin, and zinc. Amalgam is currently used in about 80 to 90 percent of tooth restorations.

It is claimed that amalgam causes or worsens MS by release of mercury which damages the immune and nervous systems. Treatment involves removal of the amalgam and replacement with gold or plastic fillings.

There is no evidence that mercury causes MS or that removal of dental amalgam improves the course of MS. Dental amalgam removal as a treatment for MS is not supported by multiple professional organizations, including the National Multiple Sclerosis Society of the United States.

Dental amalgam removal is generally well tolerated and moderately expensive.

Dietary Supplements

A wide range of compounds is included in the category of dietary supplements. Vitamins, minerals, and herbs are commonly used supplements. Other diverse compounds, including amino acids, hormones, and enzymes, are also classified as dietary supplements. In this section, dietary supplements that are popular or are relevant to MS are addressed.

Antioxidants

Free radicals are chemicals that may injure cells in the body through a process known as *oxidative damage*. Antioxidants are compounds that can decrease oxidative damage. Commonly used antioxidants include selenium and vitamins A, C, and E. Other compounds in the antioxidant category include alpha-lipoic acid, inosine, uric acid, coenzyme Q10 (CoQ10), grape seed extract, pycnogenol, and oligomeric proanthocyanidins (OPCs). Antioxidants are sometimes specifically marketed as a treatment for MS.

There are two major reasons that antioxidants are relevant to MS. First, free radicals may be involved in the pathology of MS. Myelin, the *insulation* of nerve fibers, may be injured in MS by the release of free radicals by immune cells. Also, the nerve fibers themselves, the axons, are damaged in MS through a degenerative process that may involve free radicals. Indeed, some studies indicate that oxidative damage is increased in experimental allergic encephalomyelitis (EAE), the animal model of MS, and in tissue from people with MS. The other MS-relevant aspect of antioxidants is that diets that are enriched in polyunsaturated fatty acids, which are sometimes recommended for MS (see Diets below), may cause vitamin E deficiency and supplementation with vitamin E may be needed.

Specific studies of antioxidants in MS are very limited. Studies in EAE, the animal model of MS, indicate that antioxidants may decrease disease severity. Recent studies have shown that alpha-lipoic acid and uric acid are effective therapies for EAE. Clinical studies in people with MS are currently being conducted with alpha-lipoic acid and inosine, a compound that is converted to uric acid.

Since many antioxidant compounds activate immune cells which are already excessively active in MS, further stimulation by antioxidants could potentially worsen the disease. Whether this occurs and is clinically important in MS has not been investigated. Thus, it represents a *theoretical risk*. The safety of many dietary supplements, including antioxidants, has not been determined in women who are pregnant or breast-feeding. Supplementation with antioxidants is a low-cost therapy.

Cranberry and Other Supplements Used for Urinary Tract Infections

People with MS are prone to bladder difficulties, including urinary tract infections (UTIs). Cranberry may help to prevent UTIs.

Limited clinical studies with cranberry indicate that it may prevent UTIs in some people. Specifically, beneficial effects have been found in studies of UTI prevention in women with normal bladder function. However, in limited studies of people with abnormal bladder function, which may occur in MS, cranberry was actually found to be ineffective for preventing UTIs. The ideal clinical trial with cranberry has not been done in any group of people. The evidence for two other UTI-related dietary supplements, vitamin C and bearberry (uva-ursi), is less clear than that for cranberry. Clinical studies do not provide strong support for either of these in the prevention of UTIs.

Cranberry is inexpensive and generally well tolerated. Cranberry tablets are less expensive than juice. Cranberry may interfere with blood-thinning medications, such as warfarin (Coumadin®). Long-term use of high doses may increase the risk of kidney stones and may cause gastrointestinal discomfort, loose stools, and nausea. There is insufficient information about the safety of cranberry in women who are pregnant or breastfeeding.

Echinacea and Other "Immune-Stimulating" Supplements

Echinacea and several other dietary supplements are known to activate the immune system. In some alternative medicine books, it is erroneously stated that MS is an immune disease and that, consequently, people with MS should take echinacea and other dietary supplements that stimulate the immune system. This is incorrect and *potentially dangerous* information. Since MS is characterized by excessive immune system activity, compounds that stimulate the immune system, such as echinacea, could actually *worsen* the disease.

The immune system effects of some dietary supplements have undergone limited investigation in *test-tube* or animal experiments. These studies have investigated components of the immune system that are excessively active in MS. Activation of these cells has been produced by echinacea and several other dietary supplements, including:

- Herbs: alfalfa, Asian ginseng, astragalus, cat's claw, garlic, maitake mushroom, mistletoe, shiitake mushroom, Siberian ginseng, stinging nettle

- Vitamins and minerals: antioxidant vitamins and minerals (see Antioxidants above), zinc

- Melatonin

Based on scientific evidence, these compounds pose theoretical risks to people with MS.

Ginkgo Biloba

Ginkgo biloba usually refers to the extract that is derived from the leaf of the *Ginkgo biloba* tree. Among herbs, ginkgo is one of the most extensively studied and one of the most popular.

There are several effects of ginkgo that are relevant to MS. First, it is possible that it could treat the disease itself. Ginkgo has anti-inflammatory and antioxidant effects, both of which could be therapeutic for MS. In addition, since ginkgo may improve cognitive function in people with Alzheimer's disease, it has been proposed that it may have similar effects on MS-related cognitive dysfunction.

Ginkgo has undergone limited investigation in MS. Ginkgo and related compounds decreased disease severity in some, but not all, studies in the animal model of MS. One small study of people with MS found that it may be helpful for MS attacks; however, this was *not* supported by a subsequent study that was larger and was more rigorously conducted. Thus, it does not appear to be effective for MS attacks. Whether ginkgo prevents attacks—in a way similar to interferons, glatiramer acetate, mitoxantrone, and natalizumab—has never been investigated. One preliminary study found that ginkgo may improve MS-related cognitive difficulties. Further studies are needed to determine if ginkgo has the effect of slowing the course of MS or improving MS cognitive difficulties.

Ginkgo is usually well tolerated. It may have a blood-thinning effect and thus should be avoided in people who have bleeding disorders, take antiplatelet or anticoagulant medication, or are undergoing surgery. In addition, ginkgo may provoke seizures and should be used with caution by those with seizure disorders. It may also cause dizziness, rashes, headache, and gastrointestinal complaints, including nausea, vomiting, diarrhea, and flatulence. The safety of ginkgo in women who are pregnant or breast-feeding is not known. Ginkgo is inexpensive.

St. John's Wort

St. John's wort has been used as an antidepressant for more than 2,000 years. It is so named because it blooms around the time of the feast day of St. John the Baptist (June 24). The red pigments in its buds and flowers are associated with the blood of St. John the Baptist. Depression is a relatively common symptom in people with MS.

St. John's wort may be effective for treating mild-moderate depression. In a 1996 report, a combined analysis of 23 different clinical studies involving 1,757 people reported that St. John's wort appeared to be effective for treating mild-moderate depression. Subsequently, some studies have questioned the potency of the antidepressant effect of St. John's wort. There is no evidence that St. John's wort is effective for treating severe depression. It is unclear how the effectiveness of St. John's wort compares to that of the newer antidepressants known as selective serotonin reuptake inhibitors (SSRIs), such as fluoxetine (Prozac®), paroxetine (Paxil®), and sertraline (Zoloft®).

Although St. John's wort is usually well tolerated, there are several important factors related to its use. People who are concerned they may have depression should not attempt to diagnose and treat this condition on their own. St. John's wort may worsen MS fatigue or increase the sedating effects of some medications. St. John's wort may cause a sensitivity of the skin and nerves to sunlight ("photosensitivity"), especially in those who are fair skinned. It should be avoided by women who are pregnant or breast-feeding because of possible side effects. Finally, St. John's wort may alter the levels of multiple drugs, including anticonvulsants, antidepressants, heart medications, blood-thinning medications, and oral contraceptives. St. John's wort is inexpensive.

Valerian

People with MS are prone to sleep disorders. Valerian, an herb that has been used for more than 1,000 years, may be helpful for treating insomnia. The mechanism by which valerian might produce its actions is unclear.

Several clinical studies suggest that valerian is effective for treating insomnia, but have been of variable quality. Valerian is also sometimes claimed to be effective for depression, insomnia, and muscle stiffness (spasticity). However, due to limited clinical studies, its effects on these conditions are not known.

Valerian is generally safe. It may cause sedation, which may worsen MS fatigue or increase the sedating effects of some medications. The safety of long-term use and use during pregnancy or breast-feeding has not been established. Valerian is inexpensive.

Vitamin B12 (Cobalamin, Cyanocobalamin)

Supplements of vitamin B12, also known as cobalamin or cyanocobalamin, are sometimes claimed to be effective therapies for MS. Vitamin B12 is essential for maintaining normal nervous system functioning. People with vitamin B12 deficiency, like some people with MS, have injury to the optic nerves and the spinal cord. For these and other reasons, it is sometimes concluded that vitamin B12 supplements could be effective MS therapies.

The mechanism by which nervous system injury occurs in MS is different from that associated with vitamin B12 deficiency. In addition, most people with MS have normal vitamin B12 levels. For people who have normal vitamin B12 levels, there is no evidence that vitamin B12 supplements provide any significant beneficial effects. Importantly, there is a small subgroup of people with MS who have vitamin B12 deficiency. In that case, treatment with vitamin B12 is recommended.

Vitamin B12 supplements are usually well tolerated. Rarely, vitamin B12 may cause diarrhea, rashes, and itching. Vitamin B12 is inexpensive.

Vitamin D and Calcium

Vitamin D and calcium have multiple actions in the body, including an important role in maintaining bone density. Vitamin D and calcium are relevant to people with MS for two reasons. First, people with MS are at risk for developing osteoporosis and a less severe form of decreased bone density known as osteopenia. In addition, vitamin D and calcium mildly suppress immune system function in a way that could be therapeutic for people with MS.

A possible therapeutic effect for vitamin D in MS is suggested by several studies. In the animal model of MS, disease severity is worsened by vitamin D deficiency and improved by vitamin D supplementation. Epidemiologic studies indicate that the use of vitamin D supplements is associated with a decreased risk of developing MS. Unfortunately, there is very limited clinical trial information about vitamin D and MS. A preliminary report of a small, short-term study of 11 people with MS found that treatment with a form of vitamin D did not produce significant benefits. Another study found that *calcitriol*, the active form of vitamin D, was generally safe and well tolerated in people with MS for up to 1 year—this study was not designed to determine if calcitriol had therapeutic effects in MS.

In reasonable doses, vitamin D and calcium are usually well tolerated. Calcium may interfere with the absorption of some medications (antibiotics, thyroid medication, osteoporosis medication) and minerals (iron, magnesium, zinc). In high doses, vitamin D and calcium may cause multiple side effects. Vitamin D and calcium are inexpensive.

Diets

Many diets have been proposed as effective MS therapies. For many of these diets, there is no clear underlying rationale or clinical evidence to support their use in MS. Diets for MS that are *not* supported by a strong rationale or clinical data include allergen-free diets, gluten-free diets, pectin-restricted diets, fructose-restricted diets, severely sugar-restricted diets, and diets that reduce or eliminate processed foods.

On the basis of scientific, epidemiologic, animal model, and clinical trial studies, there is suggestive evidence that diets that are low in saturated fats and high in polyunsaturated fatty acids (PUFAs) may have a therapeutic effect in MS. PUFAs include omega-3 and omega-6 fatty acids. Omega-6 fatty acids include compounds known as linoleic acid and gamma-linolenic acid. Examples of omega-3 fatty acids include eicosapentanoic acid (EPA), docosahexanoic acid (DHA), and alpha-linolenic acid (ALA). The remainder of this section will review three PUFA-related dietary approaches. The first PUFA-enriched diet that was extensively studied in MS was the Swank diet. Subsequently, several MS clinical studies evaluated the effects of supplementation with omega-6 and omega-3 fatty acids.

The Swank Diet

In the 1940s, Dr. Roy Swank developed a dietary approach that has been reported to be an effective treatment for MS. With this diet, saturated fat intake is decreased to 15 grams (g) or less daily, high-fat dairy products are excluded, frequent fish meals are recommended, and 10 to 15 g of fluid vegetable oil and 5 g of cod-liver oil is added to the daily diet.

This diet was developed due to the apparent association of dietary fat intake with MS. Specifically, early epidemiologic studies indicated that MS is less common in populations that consume relatively low levels of saturated fats and relatively high levels of PUFAs. Studies conducted subsequent to the development of the Swank diet have provided additional rationale for this type of dietary approach (see below under Supplementation with Omega-6 Fatty Acids and Supplementation with Omega-3 Fatty Acids).

There have been several reports of the initial group of people with MS who were treated with the Swank diet. In one of these reports, 134 people with MS were monitored for 34 years on the Swank diet. In the first year on the diet, the rate of MS attacks was decreased by 70 percent relative to the attack rate prior to entering the study. Unfortunately, there was no placebo-treated group in this study. As a result, the people in the study were compared to people with MS reported in the medical literature who did not receive any type of MS treatment. When this type of comparison was done, it was found that people on the diet had less frequent attacks, less progression of neurologic disability, and decreased mortality. These beneficial effects were greatest in those who adhered strictly to the diet and those who were mildly affected or were early in the course of the disease. Although these findings are encouraging, this study has significant shortcomings. As noted, there was no placebo-treated group. In addition, people who were treated were not randomly selected for treatment, and the examining clinicians and the treated patients were not "blind" to whether they were being treated. Due to these and other shortcomings, this study is not rigorous enough to provide definitive conclusions about the effectiveness of this dietary approach.

This diet is usually well tolerated. Long-term adherence to the diet may not be possible because the recommended food is not appealing. Due to the decreased meat intake in the Swank diet, people who use this dietary approach should be certain that protein intake is adequate. Although cod-liver oil, one component of this diet, is generally safe, it may rarely cause adverse effects. Cod-liver oil may have a blood-thinning effect and should be used with caution by those who take aspirin or anticoagulant medication, are undergoing surgery, or have bleeding disorders. Diabetics should also use cod-liver oil with caution. Finally, cod-liver oil contains relatively high concentrations of vitamin A, which may be toxic in doses greater than 10,000 IU. The Swank diet is inexpensive.

Supplementation with Omega-6 Fatty Acids

Supplementation with omega-6 fatty acids is an approach that increases the intake of polyunsaturated fatty acids (PUFAs). Most studies of omega-6 fatty acid supplementation have used sunflower seed oil or evening primrose oil. Other dietary supplements that contain omega-6 fatty acids include flaxseed oil, borage seed oil, black currant seed oil, and spirulina (blue-green algae).

As noted for the Swank diet (see above), epidemiologic studies indicate that a high intake of PUFAs may be associated with a lower risk of developing MS. There are other findings that support the use of a diet enriched in omega-6 fatty acids. Some, but not all, studies have shown that the blood levels of PUFAs are decreased in people with MS. In addition, scientific studies show that in the body PUFAs are converted to compounds which have anti inflammatory effects and immune system–modulating effects that, on a theoretical basis, could be therapeutic for MS.

In the animal model of MS, disease severity is worsened by deficiencies in omega-6 fatty acids and lessened by supplementation with omega-6 fatty acids. In people with relapsing remitting MS (RRMS), three placebo-controlled clinical trials have evaluated supplementation with omega-6 fatty acids. In these studies, the treated group received sunflower seed oil, which contains an omega-6 fatty acid known as linoleic acid. In two of these studies, there was a significant decrease in the duration and severity of MS attacks. In the other study, there was not a therapeutic effect. A reanalysis of these three studies, for which not all of the original data was available, showed that people with mild disability had a statistically significant decrease in progression of disability and a statistically significant decrease in attack severity and duration; people with moderate-severe disability had no significant change in disability and a statistically significant decrease in attack severity and duration. In studies of people with progressive MS, omega-6 fatty acid supplementation has not been effective. Evening primrose oil, a dietary supplement that contains an omega-6 fatty acid known as gamma-linolenic acid has not produced therapeutic effects in people with relapsing-remitting or progressive disease.

Supplementation with omega-6 fatty acids is usually well tolerated. The safety of long-term supplementation with omega-6 fatty acids has not been well studied. A concern has been raised that linoleic acid supplementation may increase the risk of some forms of cancer, but this has not been proven. Since supplementation with PUFAs may cause vitamin E deficiency, supplementation with vitamin E may be necessary. Evening primrose oil, and perhaps other gamma-linolenic acid–containing supplements (black currant seed oil, borage seed oil, spirulina), may rarely provoke seizures. Also, gamma-linolenic acid–containing supplements may have blood-thinning effects. Omega-6 fatty acid supplements may increase tri-glyceride levels and thus should be used with caution by people with elevated triglycerides. One specific supplement, borage seed oil, may contain liver toxins. The safety of black currant seed oil has not been well studied. Spirulina products may contain heavy metals, bacteria, and other contaminants. The safety of omega-6 fatty acid supplementation in women who are pregnant or breast-feeding is not known. Supplementation with omega-6 fatty acids is inexpensive.

Supplementation with Omega-3 Fatty Acids

This approach increases the intake of omega-3 fatty acids, which include eicosapentaenoic acid (EPA), docosahexaenoic acid (DHA), and alpha-linolenic acid (ALA). EPA and DHA are present in relatively high levels in fish, especially fatty fish such as salmon, Atlantic herring, Atlantic mackerel, bluefin tuna, and sardines. Dietary supplements containing EPA and DHA include fish oil and cod-liver oil. Rich sources of ALA include flaxseed oil, canola oil, and walnut oil.

The rationale for this approach is similar to that outlined for the Swank diet and supplementation with omega-6 fatty acids (see above, under The Swank Diet and Supplementation with Omega-6 Fatty Acids). In addition, immunologic studies indicate that, among the polyunsaturated fatty acids (PUFAs), the omega-3 fatty acids exert the most potent anti-inflammatory and immune-modulating effects. Also, omega-3 fatty acids appear to be important in forming and maintaining myelin, a part of the nervous system that is injured in MS.

Studies of omega-3 fatty acid supplementation in the animal model of MS are limited and conflicting. The most rigorous clinical study of this approach was a placebo-controlled trial of fish oil in people with RRMS. There was a trend for the treated group to show less disease progression, fewer attacks, and decreased attack duration, but these findings were not statistically significant. Therapeutic effects were noted in two uncontrolled studies, one with cod-liver oil, calcium, and magnesium and the other with fish oil, other dietary supplements, and dietary advice. A small study evaluated omega-3 fatty acid supplementation in combination with interferons or glatiramer acetate. People were treated with their MS medications along with either fish oil and a very low-fat diet or with olive oil and a low-fat diet. There was a trend for improved physical and emotional functioning in those taking fish oil. Both dietary interventions were associated with a decrease in relapse rate.

In the United States, the Food and Drug Administration (FDA) has classified fish oils as "generally regarded as safe." A 7-year study of fish oil use in nearly 300 people did not find any serious side effects. The long-term safety of other omega-3 fatty acid supplements is not known. Increased dietary intake of ALA may increase the risk of prostate cancer. Although fish oil supplements generally do not have a significant amount of mercury, some fish, such as shark, swordfish, and king mackerel, do contain relatively high mercury levels. Fish and flaxseed oil may have a blood-thinning effect. Fish oil may impair lung function in those who are aspirin sensitive. High doses of fish oil may increase blood sugar levels in diabetics. High doses of flaxseed oil may produce cyanide toxicity. There are potential side effects that are specifically associated with cod-liver oil (see above, under The Swank Diet). For women who are pregnant or breast-feeding, the safety of omega-3 fatty acid supplements, including fish oil, is not known. Supplementation with omega-3 fatty acids is inexpensive.

Other Types of Therapy

Feldenkrais

Feldenkrais, a type of bodywork, teaches comfortable and efficient body movements. It is claimed to improve multiple symptoms and to provide therapeutic effects for people with MS. The retraining of movements with Feldenkrais is believed to increase the efficiency and comfort of body movements. This is claimed to improve walking stability, increase strength and coordination, and decrease stress.

Feldenkrais has undergone very limited investigation in MS and other conditions. In one small study, 20 people with MS were treated for 8 weeks with either Feldenkrais or sham sessions. The treated group had significantly decreased stress and a trend for decreased anxiety relative to the sham group. This study was not rigorous enough to be conclusive.

Feldenkrais is generally safe and of low-moderate cost.

Guided Imagery and Relaxation

Guided imagery, also known as *imagery* or *visualization*, is a relaxation method, often used in combination with other relaxation methods, such as progressive muscle relaxation. It is claimed to be effective for treating a variety of symptoms including anxiety, depression, and pain. In guided imagery, an individual creates mental images that have specific effects on the body and mind.

In one published study of 33 people with MS, it was found that anxiety was decreased, but these methods had no effect on depression or other MS symptoms. Larger and more rigorous studies are needed.

Guided imagery and relaxation are usually well tolerated. Relaxation may cause or worsen muscle stiffness. Imagery may cause fear of losing control, anxiety, and disturbing thoughts, and so people with psychiatric conditions should use it with caution. Guided imagery is inexpensive.

Hyperbaric Oxygen

Hyperbaric oxygen (HBO) treatment is a form of oxygen therapy in which a person breathes oxygen under increased pressure in a specially designed chamber. It is claimed that HBO is effective for MS and many other diseases.

The oxygen content of the blood increases with the use of HBO that results in an increased amount of oxygen in different body tissues. It is believed that this is therapeutic for a variety of medical conditions.

HBO is an accepted treatment for a limited number of specific medical conditions, including burns, severe infections, and decompression sickness (due to deep-sea diving). Unfortunately, there is no strong evidence to support the use of HBO in MS and many other diseases. An early study of HBO in MS, reported in 1983, found that it was effective. However, subsequently, many clinical trials were conducted and generally found that HBO did not produce beneficial effects in people with MS. A mild improvement in bladder function was reported in a few studies. Large independent reviews of all of the published HBO and MS clinical trials were published in 1995 and 2004. Both reviews conclude that there is no consistent therapeutic effect of HBO in people with MS and that HBO should not be used to treat MS. In addition, the 2004 article, a *Cochrane Database Review*, concludes that, on the basis of existing evidence, further studies of HBO in MS are not justified.

HBO is usually well tolerated. Reversible, mild visual symptoms may occur. Rarely, HBO may cause serious side effects, including seizures, collapsed lungs, pressure injury to the ear, and cataracts. HBO is expensive.

Magnetic Field Therapy (Electromagnetic Therapy)

There are two main forms of this therapy: static, permanent magnets and pulsed electromagnetic fields. Static magnetic therapy involves the use of magnetized devices such as bracelets, belts, and mattress pads. Pulsed electromagnetic field therapy, which has been more extensively studied in MS than static magnets, uses devices that produce pulsing, electromagnetic fields at a specific frequency. In one MS study, devices with a strong, pulsing magnetic field were placed on the spine. In other studies, small devices with weak, pulsing magnetic fields were placed on the legs or specific acupuncture points.

There have been four placebo-controlled clinical trials of pulsed electromagnetic therapy in MS. Three of these have involved weak magnetic fields; one involved strong magnetic fields applied to the spine. In the study of strong magnetic fields applied to the spine, spasticity was found to be significantly decreased in the treated group compared to the placebo group. In the three studies with the weaker devices, beneficial effects on spasticity and improvement in pain, bladder function, hand function, fatigue, and quality of life were found in some studies. Given the variable findings and lack of rigor in some of these studies, further investigation is needed to clarify whether this therapy has definite beneficial effects.

Short-term use of magnetic field therapy is usually well tolerated. The long-term effects of this treatment have not been investigated. Treatment with a strong magnet on the spine may produce dizziness and a band-like sensation around the torso. The weaker devices may cause headaches. Pregnant women and people with pacemakers or other electronic medical devices should consult with their physician before using these devices. Devices with a weak magnetic field are of low-moderate cost. Devices with a strong magnetic field are for experimental use and are not generally available.

Massage

Massage, one of the oldest forms of treatment, is a form of bodywork in which soft tissue is manipulated with pressure and traction. The common forms of massage in Western countries are derived from Swedish massage, which was developed by a Swedish physician in the 19th century.

In one study of massage therapy, 24 people with MS were assigned either to a control group that received "standard medical care" or to a massage treatment group that received standard medical care in combination with twice-weekly, in-home massage therapy. Relative to the start of the study, the treatment group exhibited less anxiety and depression after the first massage session and improvement in self-esteem, body image, "image of disease progression," and social functioning at the end of the 5-week study. The results of this study are promising but not definitive. Larger studies with more well-matched groups and more rigorous study design are needed.

Massage is usually well tolerated. Minor side effects include headache, lethargy, and muscle pain. More serious side effects, such as bone fractures and bleeding into the liver, are possible but rare. Massage should be avoided or used with caution by people with the following conditions: clotted blood vessels (thrombosis), burns, skin infections, open wounds, bone fractures, osteoporosis, cancer, pregnancy, and heart disease. Massage is of low-moderate cost.

Reflexology

Reflexology is a type of bodywork in which manual pressure is applied to specific areas. These areas, which are usually on the feet but may also be on the hands and ears, are thought to correspond to specific parts of the body.

It is believed that pressure at specific reflexology sites improves energy flow to the corresponding body parts. This improved energy flow is claimed to improve health.

In one controlled study of reflexology, 71 people with MS were treated for 11 weeks with either reflexology or nonspecific massage of the calf area. Relative to the control group, the people treated with reflexology exhibited significant improvement in paresthesias, urinary symptoms, and spasticity. Larger and more rigorous studies with lower dropout rates are needed.

Reflexology is generally well tolerated. Mild side effects include fatigue, foot pain, and changes in bowel and bladder function. Reflexology should be avoided or used with caution by people with bone or joint conditions of the feet and by those with other foot conditions such as gout, ulcers, and vascular disease.

Tai Chi

Tai chi is a traditional Chinese martial art that has been prac-
ticed for centuries in China. There has been recent interest in tai chi
in some Western countries. Tai chi is characterized by a series of
body postures that are linked by slow, graceful movements.

In one study, 19 people with variable levels of MS disability were
enrolled in an 8-week tai chi program. At the end of the program,
there was improvement in walking speed and muscle stiffness, as
well as in vitality, social and emotional functioning, and ability to
carry out physical and emotional roles. Another study of 16 people
with MS used the tai chi principle of "mindfulness of movement,"
which involves developing moment-to-moment awareness of movement, breathing, and posture. Relative to the control group, which
received "current available care," the treated group did not improve
in balance but did improve in multiple MS-associated symptoms, as
assessed by patients and by their relatives. Relative to pretreatment,
the treated group improved in balance. Larger and more rigorous
studies are needed.

Tai chi is usually well tolerated. Mild side effects include strained
muscles and joints. It may worsen MS-related fatigue. It should be
avoided or used with caution by those with severe osteoporosis, acute
low back pain, significant joint injuries, and bone fractures. Tai chi is
low-moderate cost.

Yoga

Yoga is a mind-body approach that was developed in India thousands of years ago. It is derived from the Sanskrit word for *union* and
is meant to unite the mind, body, and spirit. In *hatha yoga*, one of the
more popular forms of yoga, the three main components are breathing, meditation, and posture.

In spite of yoga's popularity in some countries, there are very
limited clinical studies of its effects in MS and other diseases. There
is one well-designed, controlled trial of yoga in MS. In this 6-month

study, 69 people with MS were randomized to a control group that received no intervention or to groups that were treated with conventional exercise or yoga. Relative to the control group, the yoga and conventional exercise groups had significant decreases in fatigue on the basis of two different measures. There were no consistent effects of yoga or conventional exercise on cognitive function or mood. It is not possible to determine whether yoga's effects on fatigue were due to the result of the yoga itself or resulted from other factors, such as a placebo response or benefits from being in a social setting.

Yoga is generally safe. In the clinical trial of yoga and MS, it was not associated with any serious adverse effects. Difficult postures or vigorous exercise should be avoided or done with caution by pregnant women, people with significant heart, lung, or bone conditions, or people with heat sensitivity, fatigue, and decreased balance. Yoga is a low-cost therapy, especially when it is done in groups.

5

IIIIIIIIIIIIIIIIIIIIIIIIIIIIIIIIIIIIIIIIIIIIIIIIIIIIIIIIIIIIIIIIIIIIIIIIIIIIIIIIIIIIIIIIIIIIIIIIIIIIIIIIIIIIIIIIIIIIIIII

Practical Guidelines for Living with Multiple Sclerosis

There are many things you can do to stay as healthy as possible, take control of your life, and cope with the challenges that multiple sclerosis (MS) may bring. The disease should not be in control—*you* are in control of your life, your attitudes, your relationships, your approach to problems, your interests, and your activities. The best way to take control is to obtain information and learn more about MS.

This chapter discusses some things you should do and some things you should not do. For example, you should get more information about MS; you should make sure you have an opportunity to ask questions about the disease; you should exercise; you should try to live a normal, active life, adapting to any limitations; you should work to improve your relationships; you should express a positive attitude; and you should have regular medical assessments.

The things you should not do are actually fewer in number. For example, do not withdraw from life and friends; do not stop exercising;

do not expose yourself to a hot environment; do not try every drug, herb, therapy, and procedure that you hear about without first getting reliable information about the scientific evidence, possible benefits, and side effects; and do not feel ashamed or diminished because you have MS.

Should I Learn More About Multiple Sclerosis?

MS is a disorder of the central nervous system. Many things are known about MS, and many advances are being made. There still are a great deal of unanswered questions, but it is important to learn more about the questions that are being asked by researchers and the theories that are being tested.

The best initial source of information is the MS Society. In the United States, call 800-FIGHT-MS to reach the National MS Society, and in Canada call 800-268-7582 (see Chapter 12 for the number of the nearest office of the MS Society of Canada).

What Should Others Know About Multiple Sclerosis?

It is important for your family, friends, and coworkers to understand MS. Initially you may feel that you do not want anyone to know that you have MS. That is understandable, but it is essential to tell the people you love, and others when necessary, so that they can understand and help you deal with the disease. Most people with MS are pleased and surprised at how supportive and understanding others are when they are informed. Many people may have guessed that something was wrong but did not know what to do or say. Until they know the truth (see Chapter 7), employers may not understand your need to take time off or to rest, and they may think you are not working well. Decisions to inform should be made on an individual basis, but, in general, disclosure is a good idea.

Once family and friends are aware of your diagnosis, they might benefit from literature that would allow them to better understand MS. In particular, your family should understand your symptoms and problems so they can be helpful and supportive. This is not possible if they are unaware of your MS and how it makes you feel.

Who Can Answer My Questions?

It is important to have your concerns addressed and your questions answered. Sometimes people are afraid that they might ask too many questions or that their questions might not be clear. Make a list of the questions you want to ask. Call the MS Society or bring the questions to your physician or nurse on your next visit. You probably will find that they are questions most people ask and that they are not new to the staff. If there is no clear answer to a question, it is important to find that out as well. Each new piece of information will add to your overall understanding of MS.

What Can I Learn from Other People Who Have Multiple Sclerosis?

People with MS soon learn that it is a common neurologic disorder and that there are many others in their community who have the same disease. It often helps to talk to others who share the challenges and problems of coping with MS, but there are some cautions. *You cannot compare yourself with others in terms of the type of disease, the course, or the symptoms. Multiple sclerosis is an individual disease,* and you probably will find that the features of your MS are quite different from those of the next person. It may seem puzzling that there are so many individual patterns for the disease, but that is actually fairly common in other diseases as well. The variety of symptoms of MS is great, so the apparent variations in individuals are great as well.

One way that people with MS can benefit from each other is in self-help or support groups. These take various forms, but they usually are small groups that meet in homes or in community facilities to talk about and better understand MS. The object is always to take a positive approach and to take control over everything that you can manage so that you can help yourself and others. The MS Society has information on support groups, including how to join one or how to start one.

When Is Information Not Helpful?

Misinformation is not helpful and can cause much trouble and distress, not to mention wasted time and money. If someone says that mercury in dental fillings causes MS, check it out from those who know—staff at the MS Society, someone in the MS clinic in your area, or your physician—but do not go to the dentist and have your fillings removed. If someone tells you that ginseng cures MS, check it out. If someone says there is a doctor in a clinic somewhere who has a cure for MS, call the MS Society, not your travel agent.

What About My Activities?

People with MS should lead normal and active lives within the limitations of their symptoms. This means that we encourage activity more than rest and staying active and involved rather than withdrawing and dropping out. We want people to remain productive and working. It is understandable that symptoms and problems may make this harder for you, that doing things may take more time and energy, but it is still better to do it than not to do it.

People with MS are happiest and at their best when they live normally and carry out the activities they enjoy. There are no absolute limitations—if you feel like climbing a mountain and do not have symptoms and problems that limit you, go for it! Unfortunately, MS does cause symptoms that may limit activities to some extent.

It requires adjustment so that you can continue to do as much as you can, in the time you need, and in the way you can manage. If you work at managing your problems, coping with any limitations, and keeping a positive attitude, not only can you do many of the things in life you want to do, but also you may accomplish much more than others without MS, as they often do not use these positive skills to deal with life.

What About Exercise?

Simply put, exercise is good for everyone. When the diagnosis of MS is made, you should set about getting yourself in the best shape that you can, both mentally and physically, in order to manage any challenges that come with the disease. We all benefit from regular exercise, and it is even more important for the person with MS. If fatigue is a problem, you should arrange your exercise for times when fatigue is less bothersome, schedule it in periods with breaks, or redesign the type and pattern of exercise so that you can still do it.

In general, the best exercise is one that you enjoy so that you will still be doing it in 6 months and in 6 years. Exercise should be a lifetime habit for all of us, including people with MS, even if the exercise program needs to be modified at times. Decide what you like to do and would enjoy doing almost every day. Try to involve others in exercise as well. Exercise programs in the community have a tendency to motivate you to participate regularly; they also have an enjoyable social aspect.

Can I Overdo It?

It would seem logical to be concerned that overdoing things might cause attacks of MS and worsen the disease and that we should rest and avoid strain and work. This is *not* good advice. *There is no evidence that doing a lot, exercising, or even overdoing activities or physical exercise has any deleterious effect on MS.* True, it may make you tired for the next day or so, but there is no evidence that it worsens your MS. Some people "push through" their fatigue, which also may make them tired the next day but does no harm.

It might be tempting to blame overactivity for the development of a new attack of MS or a new symptom, especially if it happened a day or a few days later, but a careful accounting of strenuous events, stressful events, and the occurrence of attacks would show that this probably is coincidental. Do not worry about activity; be reasonable, keep active, and do what you can.

How Much Should I Rest?

Because fatigue is a major problem for many people with MS, a reasonable balance between maintaining your normal activities and taking brief rests is appropriate. People usually find their own balance of activity and rest, and in this way they keep up their activity, work, and other responsibilities.

It is important to recognize that the fatigue in MS is not "normal" tiredness that follows too little sleep or a long, hard day. The fatigue in MS is often an abnormal sensation; it is unrelated to the amount of sleep and activity and it feels different. It can occur in waves and may seem overwhelming at times. Adapting the level of activities is often successful, and some medications also may be helpful (see Chapter 3).

Do not rest too much. *Activity* is a more important watchword than rest in MS.

What About Stress?

Everyone experiences stress in their lives, and being given a diagnosis of MS is certainly stressful. Having to see yourself and your life in a different light, with greater uncertainty, is stressful. But marriage, raising children, doing our jobs, and the "daily-ness" of life also bring stress. The central point is not whether stress is present in your life (it almost always is), but your response to it. People can, and do, react differently. Some see stress as a problem to be solved. Some respond emotionally, collapsing in tears, becoming depressed, or lashing out angrily at others. Some are initially upset, but then set about overcoming or dealing with the stress. Others do not believe it is possible to deal with it and give up. It is not the stress; it is our reaction to it that makes the difference.

When people react to stress in a nonproductive way, they often state that anyone would react the same way. That actually is not true, but some people are unable to see any other way of reacting. Fortunately, by analyzing such events, you can learn how to react more positively. It is not easy and sometimes requires counseling, but a person who reacts ineffectively to stress can learn how to respond better. It does mean that you must recognize that your responses could be more productive before you can work at it or seek help.

Can I Develop Better Coping Skills?

We all have certain patterns of coping. Some of us react more intellectually to problems and stresses, while others react more emotionally. Most of us have a combination of the two; it is the balance of intellectual problem-solving responses and emotional responses that is important.

It is natural to feel upset when something stressful happens. However, it is not normal for that to be the only response. There is a point at which we must think clearly and objectively about what the stress is all about, how we can analyze it, and how we can most effectively deal with it. That combines the appropriate emotional and problem-solving aspect. You can improve these coping skills by improving their components. When a stressful event has passed, you can analyze how well you responded: whether your emotional response was appropriate and balanced, and whether the steps you took were the most effective and efficient ones for solving or dealing with the problem. Such analysis often gives you a different perspective, particularly if it is done in an honest fashion and enables you to see how you could respond more effectively the next time.

How Can I Maintain a Positive Attitude?

The most important factor in dealing with MS—or any challenge in life—is a mature, positive, and good-humored attitude whenever possible.

Some people struggle harder than others. There is no question that a positive attitude is of great importance because a negative person cannot tolerate very much adversity. Multiple sclerosis does not make you positive or negative; you already had an approach to life before you developed the disease. Multiple sclerosis can challenge your approach, your positivity, and your good humor, however, so it is important to make an even greater effort to overcome difficulties in a way that makes you feel good and improves your relationships. People like to be around those who are positive and good humored. We can understand those who are negative and turn their frustration on others, but they do not manage well, are more unhappy, and do not learn to take control of the things they can manage.

What About My Relationships?

Good relationships are helpful to all of us, and they become even more important when we have difficult challenges to deal with and overcome. One important aspect of taking control of your health and your future is to strengthen your relationships. It may seem simplistic, but it actually is one of the most important things you can do. It has a positive effect on you when you do everything you can to improve your relationships with your spouse, your children, your family, your friends, and everyone with whom you come in contact. Our relationships with others are central to our happiness and state of well-being, and it is rewarding to continue to improve them.

Should I Tell People I Have Multiple Sclerosis?

It is natural that you may have felt uncertain about telling people—even your family or close friends—when you first were told that you have MS. It is hard to recognize that something about yourself has changed, and it is worrisome to think that it may change relationships and how people regard you. Eventually you will come to recognize that you are still the same person, that the people who love you will continue to love you and support you, and that others generally are understanding and helpful. Sometimes they may try to be too helpful, as most people do not want the relationship to be altered or to be treated differently. All of these feelings, plus some embarrassment about "having an illness," make many people want to hide the diagnosis. They think "maybe if I pretend the problem doesn't exist, it won't exist."

It is a good rule to be honest and open in our relationships and interactions. Of course, like all health matters, the fact that you have MS is a private and confidential matter, so who you confide in is a personal choice. It is common to keep the information within a small circle initially, especially because everything may be calm and stable for many years. A problem begins to develop when symptoms cause difficulties that are visible to others, but they have not been made aware that you have a health problem. At that point, others may wonder, worry, and speculate about what is happening, and their speculation can be more harmful than the truth.

It also is worth considering that people feel excluded and not trusted when they are kept in the dark yet know that something is being kept secret. There are some instances when keeping a medical problem a secret can be a serious offense or can cause serious problems.

For example, you cannot lie about having a medical problem when answering questions on insurance forms or other official documents. There are only a few instances when it is proper to ask such questions, but in such instances you must answer truthfully.

What Happens When It Is Hot?

Most, but not all, people with MS find that they are heat sensitive. They notice that they become weak or dizzy, or even feel sick, in a hot bath, on a hot humid day, or in a warm environment. They also notice the opposite—they feel better and function better when it is cooler, when they are swimming in cool water, or when they move from a warm room to a cool room.

Remyelinated and partially damaged nerve fibers may function less well when body temperature is elevated and, conversely, the nerves function better when temperature is lowered. This tends to be a transient phenomenon that does not produce a lasting effect. However, it can produce marked weakness, and people often describe themselves as feeling like a "dishrag" or "wiped out" on a hot day. This response to heat was once the basis of the *hot bath test*, which was used as a test for MS before modern diagnostic tests were available. Although it is suggestive of MS, it is not accurate enough to be an important test.

You may wonder whether becoming weak in a hot environment will make the disease worse, but the phenomenon is transient and disappears as soon as you cool off. We do recommend that you avoid a warm environment whenever possible because you will feel less well, function less well, and have more symptoms when it is very warm. Air conditioning often is required in summer months to maintain reasonable temperature control and is considered medically necessary for tax purposes (a letter from your physician is needed). Cool drinks are also helpful—get in the habit of carrying one with you. The fluids will help your bladder and bowel function as well! Avoiding sunbathing, saunas, and hot tubs is strongly advised.

Should I Change My Diet?

The dietary approach to the management of MS has a long history. It is difficult to perform clinical trials on diets, but there was interest and some suggestion of a positive response from studies of diets that are low in animal fats (essentially a low-cholesterol diet) and with a supplement of a vegetable oil such as sunflower seed oil or evening primrose oil. A few of these studies showed some positive benefit; one large study showed no benefit. There also was some suggestion that people with early and mild disease benefit the most. Many people use the simple approach to diet of lowering the amount of animal fat and supplementing it with a vegetable oil because it is a healthy diet and everyone in the family can potentially benefit from it. Many more complex diets have been recommended in MS, which have little logic or justification and are so complicated that people give them up after a short time.

The most important points are to stick to a balanced, healthy diet, maintain normal weight, and limit your intake of animal fat. This is a good dietary recommendation for everyone.

Should I Sleep More?

How much sleep you need is based on your own normal pattern. Some people require 8 or 9 hours a night, whereas others require only 5 or 6 hours. The average is 7½ hours of sleep, and the measure of effectiveness is how rested you feel in the morning. You should not change your sleep pattern because you have MS. Since fatigue is a major problem for many people, there is a tendency to think that you will be less fatigued if you sleep more. However, even with normal or greater sleep hours, you will still tend to feel tired during the day if fatigue is due to MS. Surprisingly, oversleeping often makes people feel more tired. It is worth remembering that many factors can decrease the quality of sleep, including alcohol and many drugs.

What If I Need Surgery?

The answer to this question is simple. If you need surgery and there are good indications for surgery, you should have it. If you do not need surgery, you should not have it. This is a good rule whether you have MS or not. There does not appear to be any increased risk to people with MS who undergo surgery. In the past, there was concern that the stress of surgery might precipitate MS attacks, but the number of attacks of MS that occur in those circumstances is the same as that which would be expected in an average population of people with the disease, and no more. This relates to the previous point that there is little evidence that stressful events precipitate attacks of MS, whether they involve surgery, anesthesia, trauma, or major life events. The most important rule is to be assured that surgery is truly indicated and necessary.

Is Pregnancy a Risk?

The relationship between MS and pregnancy is now fairly well understood. Pregnancy does not appear to increase the incidence of attacks of MS; in fact, some data suggest that the likelihood of an attack of MS decreases by up to 70 percent during this period. However, there is an increased number of episodes of symptoms or attacks in the 6 months following delivery than would be expected in a 6-month period. Those episodes should be treated and managed like any other episode of MS. Pregnancy has no long-term effects on disability or disease progression.

Two other aspects of pregnancy and child rearing must be considered. First, there is a small, but real, genetic risk for MS in a family—in the range of 2 to 5 percent for a first-degree relative. This is greater than the risk in the normal population, but it clearly is low. More significantly, raising a child is a life-long responsibility, and people with MS must recognize that their health during the time that they will need to carry out this responsibility may be uncertain. For example, one cannot predict health status in 10 years. This probably is the major factor that governs the decision about having a child. Recognizing the risks and problems, each couple must determine for themselves this very personal decision. An excellent resource on this topic is the book *The Disabled Woman's Guide to Pregnancy and Birth* (see Additional Readings).

Will Multiple Sclerosis Affect My Sex Life?

Because MS affects the central nervous system and the nerves that control various functions in the body, the complex and sensitive control system for sexual function also can be affected. Early in the disease there may be no physical effect on sexual function, but the enjoyment of sex may be affected by your emotional state. Worries, depression, or altered feelings about yourself can affect your relationship with others and the normal emotions associated with sexuality. Thus, sexual function may be affected by psychologic factors, and this possibility needs to be considered. More often there is a physiologic basis for the difficulties, which often are seen in conjunction with bladder and bowel symptoms. For men, the most common problem is achieving or maintaining an erection, which can be helped by medication such as sildenafil citrate (Viagra®). Women may experience decreased vaginal lubrication, which can be accommodated by synthetic lubricating products, such as Astroglide®.

What About Driving?

Driving is only a problem when symptoms or limitations make it risky or unacceptably difficult. Vertigo, double vision, or a temporary loss of vision would not permit you to drive safely. Problems with leg weakness or incoordination limit rapid and accurate use of brake and accelerator pedals and make driving unsafe. It may be possible to return to driving when symptoms improve, but it is wise to depend on the assessment of your physician when there is any question about this. Most rehabilitation facilities can assess whether a person can drive safely.

When a problem is more long standing and renders driving unsafe, it may be possible to adapt the controls on the vehicle to allow a person to drive. The most common adaptation is that foot pedals are converted to manual control.

Although a person may be anxious to continue driving and willing to take some chances, feeling that they are "all right to drive," greater consideration must be given to others who may be at risk, including passengers and pedestrians.

Should I Move?

Some people with MS ask if it would be helpful if the moved to another area because they have read that the incidence of MS varies in different parts of the world, that it is more common in temperate climates, and that it is rare in very hot climates, such as near the equator. The answer is no. In fact, they might find the heat a problem because it tends to make people with MS feel worse. We also believe that the geographic patterns of MS incidence probably have other explanations, and there is no evidence that moving to another area once you have the disease will help.

Will I Be Different?

It is natural to wonder how MS will change you. Young people see themselves as healthy and do not visualize themselves with a serious disease. When you are given a diagnosis of a medical condition, it is natural to begin to think of yourself differently, and you may have to readjust your self-concept. You are still *you*, but it requires you to see that a different element has entered your life.

Many things change as you go through life—some good, some not so good. What is necessary is a positive approach to challenges and determination to move ahead.

What About Other Questions I May Have?

We could not possibly anticipate all the questions you may have about what to do and not to do, but we have tried to anticipate the most common questions. You will have many more, and they should be asked of your physician, other health-care professionals, or staff at the MS Society. It is always better to ask a question even if you are uncertain about exactly how to ask it or if you think it sounds "silly" than to wonder or worry in silence.

We recommend the book *Multiple Sclerosis: The Questions You Have—The Answers You Need* as a more detailed guide to many of your questions (see Additional Readings).

6

||||||||||||||||||||||||||||||||||||||||||||||||||||||||||||||||||||||||||||||||||||||||||||||||||||||||||||||||

Coping with Multiple Sclerosis

Being diagnosed with multiple sclerosis (MS) can create turmoil in every area of a person's life. In some ways, life will never be quite the same again. Even in the absence of impairment, the worry—or effort to camouflage worry—is always there. The diagnosis often precipitates a roller coaster ride of emotions, including fear, optimism, despair, and hope. The time following diagnosis can be challenging and confusing. This chapter will help you to bring perspective to the emotional turmoil and help you think about ways to ease the distress and continue with your life.

The Crisis of Diagnosis

People have a variety of reactions to hearing the diagnosis of MS for the first time. Some experience a combination of fear and panic when first confronted with the news. These feelings may quickly be replaced by denial, a refusal to believe that this could possibly be happening. "There must be some mistake!" is an almost universal reaction to the diagnosis, often followed quickly by feelings of anger and resentment. Lisa's story provides an example of some of these feelings. When asked about her initial experience with the diagnosis of MS, Lisa (then 19 years old), replied:

> *I was having a multitude of symptoms that I didn't understand, such as numbness in my feet. I was having trouble feeling the ground when I was walking. I couldn't see very well out of my left eye—it was almost like looking through an oily film. A whole bunch of odd things were happening that I didn't understand. When I finally got the diagnosis, I was really scared. I didn't know what MS was or what would happen to me. I was afraid of the whole thing.*

> *Later I was angry—very angry. Then I decided there was no way I could really have this disease. In fact, my parents and I were second guessing the doctors—going from one to another asking what was wrong with me. All I could think of was that can in the grocery store that you throw your loose change into—you know, the one with the picture of someone in a wheelchair. It was probably a good year before I even started to accept the fact that I have MS. There was no way I could have it—I'm too active and I do so many things. And I can't stop doing them.*

The diagnosis actually brings a sense of relief for some people, especially those who were beginning to wonder if they were "going crazy" or if the symptoms were "all in the mind." These fears are sometimes reinforced by physicians who, in the absence of clear physical abnormalities, believe that emotional problems may be causing imaginary or exaggerated symptoms. A small study by Loveland (National MS Society, Health Services Research Report, 1993) found that women presenting with early symptoms of MS were significantly more likely than men to get this type of response from their doctors, and that men's descriptions of physical symptoms generally were given more credence by their physicians.

Relief is also experienced by those who imagined a more distressing, or perhaps fatal, explanation for their symptoms, such as cancer.

Freed from the fears of a malignant tumor, they feel confident that the symptoms they are experiencing can be successfully managed.

Jim, who was diagnosed with MS in 2004 after a frustrating search for some answers, spoke about fear and relief at finally learning his diagnosis:

It took me a year to get a diagnosis. I was scared to death when I heard "MS." I didn't even know what MS was. But I was also relieved. When you're used to not having a label for all the strange things that are going on and suddenly the problem is identified for you, that alone is a relief—all this finally has a name.

Regardless of the initial emotional response, the diagnosis of MS creates a crisis for the individual and the entire family. The person who has been diagnosed may experience a sense of isolation despite efforts of family members to offer support. Lisa mentioned this experience:

Even though people wanted to help, I was the one who had to learn to live with it and had to learn what I needed to do to live with it. You have to make your choice of how you're going to live your life. You have to do it because it's your disease and nobody can do it for you or make it go away.

Family members are also immersed in their own concerns about the future and the impact that MS will have on their lives. The positive aspect of this type of crisis (if you can even imagine one) is that it provides an opportunity to assess future plans and a powerful motivation to take actions that support those plans. There is an opportunity to affirm the values and strengths of the individual and the family and all the good things that remain intact in spite of MS. In order to go forward, it is important to know that you can successfully move through the difficult emotions and continue to pursue your goals and dreams. A professional counselor—such as a psychologist or social worker—can be a helpful ally to the person with MS and family members in working toward a positive outlook for the future.

The Adjustment Process

The initial variable reactions to the diagnosis of MS inevitably give way to a feeling of deep sadness. This is related to the addition of a serious chronic illness to one's identity and self-image. Chronic illness forces each person to confront the frailty and vulnerability of the human condition in a personal and immediate way. One also faces the painful reality of society's negative attitudes about disease and disability. This process involves grieving for your former self-image and integrating the realities of MS into one's identity. Sadness, anger at the disease, and self-absorption are also experienced during this time.

Grieving is necessary for a person to move forward, just as it is following the loss of a loved one. Unlike the grieving we associate with death, the grieving process in chronic illness tends to ebb and flow with the symptoms and physical changes that occur over time. Grief may be postponed, but it can never be totally avoided. Sometimes these feelings may be channeled inappropriately, such as anger at one's spouse or children or at health professionals who cannot cure the illness. It is important for everyone involved to understand this grieving process and to communicate their caring and support.

The period of intense grieving may last from a few weeks to several months, with gradually diminishing intensity. As it subsides, at least for the time being, one can again begin to focus on and enjoy special relationships and daily activities. Ideally, there is a gradual acknowledgment of the permanence of MS in one's life, while maintaining a sense of continuity between the past and the future as well as a commitment to maximizing your quality of life.

Depressive feelings are to be expected as part of the initial grieving process or in response to subsequent changes or losses imposed by the illness. Over the course of the disease, however, individuals with MS are at greater than average risk for depression. They need to be able to recognize when some kind of treatment intervention would be beneficial. Symptoms of significant depression include ongoing and pervasive sadness, loss of interest in or enjoyment of important activities and relationships, feelings of hopelessness and despair, sometimes including suicidal feelings or thoughts, and changes in sleeping and eating patterns. Intervention is recommended if any of these symptoms continue for an extended period of time or seem to be worsening. It is important to realize that relief from depression is readily available. Counseling and/or antidepressant medication are very successful in relieving its symptoms. Seeking help for this problem demonstrates an understanding of its significance, not personal weakness or deficiency.

Jim comments on his experience with depression:

I was pretty depressed, so I went to see a psychologist. She was connected with a rehabilitation facility, so her primary interest was working with people who are chronically ill or disabled to help them find comfortable ways of living and thinking about themselves. It was a perfect match because that's just what I needed at that point.

One hallmark of MS that must be addressed as part of the adjustment process is its unpredictability. When several focus groups were held by the National MS Society to identify what aspects of the disease people found most troubling and challenging, the resounding answer was the unpredictability of the disease course and the uncertainties related to future ability/disability. Questions that almost everyone faces include: what symptoms and impairments might occur, when will new symptoms appear, when will they go away, or will they go away? Amy, who was diagnosed 8 years ago, addressed this issue:

I think not knowing what will happen is the hardest thing for people when they're diagnosed with MS. They totally freak out and wonder "what's this disease going to do to me?" They have to realize that what happens to someone else is not necessarily going to happen to them. And if it does, well, you will have to deal with it.

Flexibility is a key element in living with the unpredictability of MS. Goals need to be assessed and revised, with a "plan for the worst, hope for the best" outlook. A college student named Leslie was pursuing a career in horticulture, which necessitated spending a fair amount of time in greenhouses. Her early symptoms included heat sensitivity, with temporary blurred vision and extreme fatigue when she was exposed to warm temperatures. Although this problem remitted, any future recurrence would have prevented Leslie from performing her job. After careful thought, she switched to teaching, an occupation that heat sensitivity or most other possible MS symptoms would not prevent her from continuing. Similarly, the purchase of a new home should involve consideration of issues of mobility and accessibility. Many people with MS are not significantly bothered by problems with walking. However, since mobility impairment is a problem at some point for a fair number of people with MS, it is simply good planning to consider this possibility when choosing a home, even while being reasonably optimistic that serious walking difficulties will not occur.

Coping Strategies

Coping strategies reflect an individual's personality and usual style of interfacing with people and events. By adulthood, strategies have been selected and refined through an unconscious process; most of us do not consciously choose and evaluate our coping mechanisms. However, it becomes important to look at those coping styles critically so that they can be boosted when necessary and modified or discarded when they are counterproductive. The following are examples of two types of strategies.

Denial

Denial is ignoring or minimizing the seriousness of the situation. We all engage in denial about the moment-to-moment possibility of accidental death. Intermittent denial may be useful in the early stages of adapting to MS because it enables people to deal with the immediate symptoms they are experiencing without having to contemplate all the possible problems that may occur in the future. Denial is *not* useful if these potential problems are ignored when making important life-planning decisions such as buying an accessible home or making careful career decisions. One of the most serious consequences of continued denial is avoidance of disease-modifying therapy. The availability of interventions that can have a favorable impact on the disease course for many people with MS is a very positive factor supporting hope for the future.

Denial can also interfere with obtaining optimal health care. Yes, a bladder infection may indicate underlying MS pathology and should be evaluated in light of that possibility. The numbness and tingling in your fingers may not be carpal tunnel syndrome, which is commonly associated with extensive computer use. Acknowledgment of your symptoms and paying proper attention to them will ensure that the physicians involved in your health care will provide you with the treatments you need and will not perform surgeries (e.g., for carpal tunnel syndrome or herniated disks) or prescribe treatments that are unnecessary or even harmful.

Intellectualization

Intellectualization is focusing on available factual information to the exclusion of feelings and other psychologic issues. A certain amount of intellectualization makes it possible for people to learn about the disease, assess its impact on their daily lives, and make use of their problem-solving abilities to meet the challenges imposed by MS. Intellectualization becomes excessive when it consumes enormous amounts of energy; some people expend so much effort collecting and analyzing information that they have little or no energy left to deal with their emotional reactions to the disease or with the feelings and reactions of those around them.

Looking at these two examples, the strengths and weaknesses inherent in some coping strategies can be seen. Denial is useful in allowing a person to get on with his or her life, but it is detrimental if it interferes with obtaining optimal treatment or with life-planning issues. Intellectualization is useful in obtaining essential information, but it is harmful when it is used as a means to block feelings about the disease that should be expressed. The blocking of emotional awareness and expression can interfere with long-range coping efforts.

Interpersonal difficulties may arise when two people who live together and must cope with MS have conflicting coping styles. A person who copes by talking through feelings and events or by reading all the literature on MS may encounter resistance and even anger from a partner who is trying desperately to maintain denial as a way of dealing with the disease. In some situations, counseling is useful to help a couple recognize each other's coping styles and provide mutual support. An excellent resource on this topic is *Multiple Sclerosis: A Guide for Families* (see Additional Readings).

Educate Yourself About Multiple Sclerosis

While some individuals are more inclined than others to seek information about something that is stressful to them, one of the most effective things a person with MS or a family member can do to facilitate adjustment to MS is to learn about the disease—what to expect and what can be done to relieve physical symptoms and promote psychologic health. People with MS have indicated in National MS Society surveys that information about the disease and its effects is their most important need. Education about MS is available through a number of sources, primarily MS health-care providers and the U.S., Canadian, and other national MS Societies (see Resources).

Keep in mind, however, that adults can choose to learn in a variety of ways and may choose to do so in different settings or at different times. For some, devouring every available piece of written material is the most desirable strategy. These individuals compare different sources of information, analyzing and sorting varied opinions, to create a personal perspective. The result is a sense of "ownership" of the information and its gradual integration into personal philosophy and decisions about day-to-day activities. Other people prefer a group setting that provides opportunities for the immediate testing of new ideas and feedback from peers and/or professionals.

Such group educational programs are widely available through the U.S., Canadian, and other national MS Societies. The National MS Society in the United States has a mail program called "Knowledge Is Power" for people who have been recently diagnosed with MS. The program consists of a series of modules on topics of interest sent on a predetermined schedule to people who request this service. This mail series can be obtained by calling 1-800-FIGHT-MS. These publications are also available in Canada (416-922-6065).

Another component of the educational process relates to reports of possible treatments or "the cure" for MS. Given the variability and unpredictability of the illness over time, it is not surprising that diverse therapies have been heralded as having a significant impact on MS. When symptoms remit—as they frequently do quite naturally over the course of the disease—whatever treatment or activity is being used at the time is given credit for the improvement. Since dramatic improvement and long periods of remission are common occurrences in MS, even without any therapy, it is important to be prudently skeptical when evaluating therapies that claim to be of benefit. Only those treatments that have been evaluated for safety and efficacy in carefully designed and controlled scientific studies provide documentation of benefit. Other therapies, generally outside the usual medical interventions and called "complementary" or "alternative" therapies, should also be carefully evaluated. (see Chapter 4). Some of these claim a boost to the immune system and are not appropriate for people with MS, who already have an overly active immune system. Any non–physician-prescribed therapy that claims to reduce MS disease activity or any therapy that claims to cure MS should be avoided. *Alternative Medicine and Multiple Sclerosis* is a comprehensive guide to this topic (see Additional Readings).

Choosing Your Health-Care Providers

The choice of health-care providers is a critical decision relative to long-term management issues. People with MS generally have a normal or nearly normal life expectancy, and management of the disease is a lifelong process. The physician who manages the symptoms and disease course will interact with the other physicians involved in your health care, such as your internist, gynecologist/obstetrician, cardiologist, or any other medical specialist whose services you might require during your lifetime. Members of your chosen health-care team will also provide you on an ongoing basis with information that you will need to make important life decisions relating, for example, to job choices, family planning, or the selection of an MS treatment option. Choose your health-care providers carefully. Investigate your physician's board certification (neurology, family practice, or internal medicine), experience with MS, hospital or medical center affiliation, and reputation in the community. In most cases, you will need to have a relationship with an internist or family physician to monitor your general health and serve as your "primary care provider" and a neurologist to manage your MS. The local chapter (United States) or division (Canada) of the MS Society, as well as other national MS societies, can suggest physicians in the community who have experience in the management of MS or, if none is available locally, they will identify MS specialists within the broader geographic region.

Support Networks

Family and friends provide the major support for the person with MS. Their caring and concern are vital, especially during the difficult times following diagnosis or when a flare-up of symptoms occurs.

A "sorting out" of friends and relatives may be necessary because not all people with a close relationship are able to be supportive in the same way. One person may be comfortable listening to concerns and providing emotional support, while another may find it easier to assist with more concrete activities, such as a ride to the doctor's office. Another friend or relative may be a great problem solver, helpful in finding solutions or identifying resources in troublesome situations. At the same time, a person's ability to help should not be too narrowly or rigidly determined, especially without discussing it with him or her. It is important for all those who provide support to know how important their contributions are to the person with MS.

People with MS may find it especially helpful to talk with others who have the disease. This interaction will help to demonstrate that people with MS do indeed continue productive and satisfying lives despite the intrusion of the disease. A physician or other health-care provider may be able to provide the name and phone number of someone who is willing, even eager, to talk about his or her personal experiences with MS.

Many chapters of the National MS Society have "peer support" programs that train selected individuals with MS to be helpful to people who have questions about the disease. They are available to answer questions, discuss issues, and relate their personal MS successes and failures. In some areas, the peer is available for a telephone conversation; in other areas, the person may also be available at the local MS center on certain days. Amy commented on her experience with a peer support person:

> *Having that one-on-one interaction, having someone to talk to who understands, who has gone through similar experiences—that was really important to me. She was a source of strength and kept helping my self-image to stay in shape.*

Some people find a group setting most helpful because they can benefit from the experiences of a number of people with MS. Group members also feel good about the group interaction and support, which is much like a family support network. In an MS support group, MS temporarily feels "normal" because it is the common experience of all members. This normalization of MS is extremely supportive of the overall adjustment process. Instead of feeling isolated, the person in a support group sees MS as one component of a full and diverse life, which can be managed with an understanding of the disease, support of family, friends, health professionals, and peers with MS. Some support groups are led by a counseling professional, such as a psychologist or social worker, while others are "self-help" and are led by one of the group members.

To find a support group near you, or perhaps a telephone group, call 1-800-FIGHT-MS in the United States and 1-800-268-7582 in Canada.

Disclosure

Disclosure about one's illness—whether to family members and friends, new acquaintances, or employers and colleagues—is a significant issue for most people living with MS. Many people are uncertain how much information they want or need to disclose, especially because there often is no visible impairment and some of the symptoms caused by the illness can easily be attributed to a less serious cause. Considerations about disclosure at the workplace are discussed in Chapter 7.

The first and most important group or people to consider are your family members. They are the easiest to make recommendations about, but sometimes the most difficult group to tell. Close family members need to know about your MS—what to expect and what they can do to help. In general, parents, siblings, and other close adult relatives should be told calmly and directly about the diagnosis. They need to begin learning what MS is and what is known about your prognosis and any limitations.

Children also should be told about the diagnosis. Even very young children are aware when something is wrong and tend to imagine the worst possible scenario. They need to be given some concrete information about the disease that they can relate to and understand (e.g., that Mommy will be extra tired sometimes, may have trouble walking, or will need to hurry to the toilet). They also need to be reassured that Mommy is not going to die and that she will be able to take care of them. Children need to know that, although the parent may not be able to be as physically active as before, the family will work together to solve any problems that arise. Parents should also explain that no one can "catch" MS the way a cold can be caught from another person, that the children did not cause the MS, and that they have no control over making it better or worse. Parents tend to underestimate the impact of MS on their children; they are at least as affected by their parents' emotional state and the emotional climate within the household as they are by any physical limitations imposed by illness. *Multiple Sclerosis: A Guide for Families* provides a comprehensive discussion of this topic (see Additional Readings).

What to tell friends and acquaintances may need to be determined on a case-by-case basis. How much you choose to tell will depend very much on the relationship you have with another person. Informing your friends will allow them to provide the emotional support you need and will relieve you of energy-consuming efforts to conceal the problem.

Disclosure also is an issue for people who are dating. When is the best time to tell, and how much should be revealed? As with other questions about MS, no single answer suits every individual or situation. In general, you have no obligation to talk about your MS before extending or accepting an invitation for a date. Nor should you feel any need to discuss MS before you have decided whether you like a person. Once you have decided that a relationship is worth pursuing, the following guidelines may be helpful:

- Remember that secrets and half-truths do not make a firm foundation for a healthy relationship.

- Think about when you would like to know important health-related information about the other person.

- Keep in mind that revealing your MS may become increasingly difficult as your investment in the relationship increases.

Wellness Orientation

In contrast to a *disease orientation*, which focuses on minimizing the impact of the chronic disease on all aspects of your life, a *wellness approach* looks at achieving the positive state of maximal health despite the presence of a chronic illness. Jones and Kilpatrick, in the *Families in Society Journal* (May 1996), propose a definition of wellness as the state of harmony, energy, positive productivity, and well-being in an individual's mind, body, emotions, and spirit. This model encompasses interpersonal relationships as well as relationships with the environment, the community, and society in general. The wellness orientation is comprehensive in its promotion of mind-body unity within the individual, as well as integration of the individual within the community and society as a whole.

A practical example of a wellness orientation is the practice of aerobic and general conditioning exercises, which have an orientation different from that of traditional physical therapy designed primarily to address disease-imposed impairments. Nutritional programs designed for general health (e.g., the prevention of heart disease and certain forms of cancer) go beyond traditional dietary measures that target specific MS-related problems such as constipation and urinary infections. Resources in this area include *Living with Multiple Sclerosis: A Wellness Approach and Alternative Medicine and Multiple Sclerosis* (see Additional Readings).

Practices such as yoga, meditation, and tai chi also fall within the wellness concept and are sometimes categorized as "complementary therapies" that work along with—rather than against or in place of—traditional medical therapy (see Chapter 6). Lisa again comments on her experiences, focusing on wellness behaviors:

> *I learned to watch fats and learned more about what I should eat. Now when I finish school, I usually go straight to the swimming pool and exercise for 30 to 40 minutes.*

In following a wellness approach, it is important to remember that you cannot directly impact the disease process through health-promoting behaviors. People must recognize that their control over MS is limited and that the disease may become active in spite of the health practices they have initiated. You should feel good about the wellness activities they pursue in order to enhance their general health and well-being, but not feel guilty or blame yourself when a relapse occurs. Although a wellness approach cannot control the unpredictable nature of MS, it can enable you to improve your health and devise creative ways to continue activities that are satisfying and enjoyable.

Similarly, people often believe that they can control their MS if they simply try hard enough to "fight" it. Those who engage in this kind of thinking tend to experience a sense of failure when the disease worsens. Assuming this kind of personal responsibility for disease progression is both harmful and self-defeating. Your energy— emotional and otherwise—is better channeled into pursuing wellness, always recognizing that the goal is an overall improvement in general health rather than control of the disease process.

People who struggle to control their MS sometimes feel that they are losing the battle or "giving up" if they begin to use an assistive device. These devices actually extend your abilities by conserving energy, promoting safety, and reducing effort. For example, those who fatigue easily or struggle to be ambulatory with a cane or crutches will find that their activities become severely limited. All their energy is used simply to get from one place to another, leaving little or no effort to do or enjoy whatever activity had been planned. Struggling to get to the supermarket may mean that there is no energy left to shop. People with MS should use whatever techniques, tools, or devices are available to maximize and extend their activities and opportunities. Someone who is comfortable walking for short distances may choose to use a motorized scooter on a trip to an amusement park, shopping mall, or museum. A worker in a large office who normally uses a cane might also choose to use a scooter to conserve energy and enhance productivity. The effective use of assistive devices is an important extension of the wellness philosophy. They should be seen as a means of maintaining a full, productive, and enjoyable life rather than as a symbol of defeat.

Children with MS

Although MS is considered an adult disease, it is estimated that there are between 10,000 and 20,000 children and teens with MS, or pre-MS symptoms, in the United States. This relatively rare situation presents special challenges to the family, who may feel isolated with the diagnosis in a child, and facing challenges very different from the adult MS population.

Establishing the diagnosis of MS in a child or teen can be fraught with even more difficulty than with an adult. The child is generally seen by a pediatric neurologist, who is not accustomed to seeing this disease in children. In addition, there are non-MS conditions in children that make it difficult to sort out. As a result, months or years may go by before a diagnosis is established. Once a diagnosis of MS is made, issues for the child and family are also different. Parents worry about how they might have contributed to this diagnosis (not at all), and about the future of their child with a progressive disease, who will most likely outlive them. There is also the concern about normal childhood and teenage development and milestones. How will peers react, what about educational goals, and what will be the impact on critical social relationships?

The National Multiple Sclerosis Society (The Society) has established six regional "Pediatric MS Centers of Excellence" that provide services unique to this population, and there are MS centers which address children's needs across Canada as well. At the U.S. centers, patients are seen by a team that includes both a pediatric and adult neurologist, so that the pediatric disease skills and MS expert skills can complement each other. Rehabilitation, psychosocial, and other professional services are available through each of these centers, as well as care coordination. An annual visit to one of these centers may be sufficient, with care during the intervals being provided by local healthcare professionals with guidance from the pediatric center.

Perhaps one of the most important areas for these children/teens is intervention with school personnel. Whether care is sought from one these centers or elsewhere, contact with the school is often critical. Potential cognitive dysfunction needs to be addressed, as do physical ramifications.

There is a tendency for schools to recommend schooling at home with tutors. Most children with MS can and should be maintained in their schools, and every effort should be made to support this, as appropriate. The Society's six pediatric MS centers have staff to facilitate this, and Society chapters can provide additional help.

Additionally, the National Multiple Sclerosis Society and the Multiple Sclerosis Society of Canada have a multifaceted program to support families in this situation, which includes information, networking with other families, and telephone counseling.

Cultural Sensitivity

Although the major cultural orientation in the United States and Canada is Anglo-Saxon, and in Canada French as well, families from diverse backgrounds will experience the distressing news of an MS diagnosis. While some commonality exists across cultures, it is important to recognize that real differences exist that impact upon reaction to the diagnosis and ability to provide support. For example, in some Latino groups, the family may be viewed as "cursed," indicating bad behavior deserving of punishment. In other cultures, a diagnosis of MS or other chronic illness suggests weakness on the part of the person diagnosed. These issues are too diverse and complex to address here, but it is important to recognize that reactions and behavior outside of the mainstream may have understandable explanations within a cultural context, and need to be understood by friends, family, and health-care professionals.

Parting Thoughts

Amy relates her personal philosophy:

If I had never had MS, I would never have traveled the way I did. I took a year off after I was diagnosed and traveled all around Europe. I decided I was going to do things while I could because I didn't know when something might be taken away from me. And I think one thing I've learned from MS is to do things while I can. It's a lesson for everyone. We should all live each day to the fullest, because we never know when something might happen to take it away.

Jim relates what gets him through:

I would say that I have a lot of support from my family and friends. That probably helped me through. I had quite a few conversations, talks, heart-to-heart discussions with different people, and that helped me quite a bit. Also, I'm somewhat religious and that helped.

Mary speaks about giving up denial:

I am not crazy. I have this disease, I have done nothing to deserve it, and there is nothing I can do about having it. I just have to begin to take each day, one at a time, do my best, and accept whatever comes. The sheer honesty of admitting that I have an illness is a great weight off my mind.

I am more attentive to details in my life, and more willing to do what my body tells me to do, instead of fighting against it. I have found a new calm I had not known before.

A religious or spiritual orientation has been linked with successful coping in a number of studies. It seems that religion helps some people find meaning in their illness, or at least put it into a meaningful context. Amy also refers to spirituality, as well as her own personal characteristics, as a support:

Since I grew up in a single parent household, I always had to draw on my own resources. So I worked really hard on that—and on my own sense of spirituality. I just had to—I've always depended on myself. I've always demanded a lot from myself and I guess I just drew it from within.

Amy refers to a key aspect of the coping process—a person's inner strengths. With an adult-onset disease, coping strategies have already been tested in other areas, creating a base on which to build. These strengths surface as the sense of crisis recedes. Amy has more advice for dealing with MS and with life in general.

Another thing is to laugh—to have a sense of humor. Don't take things so seriously. If you don't have a sense of humor, it's all for naught, you know. Life is too short. It can just really drag you down if you let it—you can't let that happen. Just try to take things one day at a time. One day at a time and "slow is fast enough," you don't really have to be in that much of a hurry. Take your time and take it easy and don't be afraid to ask for help.

7

‖‖

Employment Issues and Multiple Sclerosis

Most of us spend the majority of our waking hours at work and have a serious personal investment in and commitment to employment-related activities. Our self-image and identity often are closely tied to our occupation or professional status. One of the first questions asked when getting to know someone is "What kind of work do you do?" From a practical perspective, the income we receive as wages is necessary to purchase goods and services to maintain our particular lifestyle. Work that is not associated with direct financial remuneration—such as parenting, homemaking, and volunteer activities—also contributes to self-definition but usually without the lifestyle consequences. These activities, however, *will* have a financial impact if they must be replaced by the paid work of others. Given all of these factors, it is not surprising that anything that potentially threatens the ability to continue employment or other productive and rewarding activity generates concern and anxiety. A diagnosis of multiple sclerosis (MS) certainly presents this kind of distressing situation.

The good news is that most people who discover that they have MS can and should continue working after receiving their MS diagnosis. The disease-modifying immunomodulating drugs may help you to continue your employment status, although this factor has not been systematically studied. We do know that many people with the relapsing-remitting form of MS (attacks and remissions) experience fewer and less serious flare-ups when taking one of these therapies. Symptoms experienced during a flare-up of the disease may or may not interfere with your ability to function at work, and this will need.to be examined each time a relapse occurs.

Exacerbations may interfere with your usual work activities, but these episodes occur only on the average of one to two per year in the relapsing-remitting form of the disease. Progressive MS may require some changes in work activity, but disease limitations usually appear at a slow enough pace to allow for necessary modifications. It is important to be open with your employer about changes or adaptations you need in the work environment or routine that will allow you to continue to be fully productive. Employers already have made changes that are linked to prevention of disability, such as ergonomic desk chairs and hands-free headsets for the telephone. When put in this context, it likely will be easier for your employer to understand the benefit to productivity and the win-win situation for both of you.

A person with a recent diagnosis of MS may not quickly or easily arrive at a comfort level with the disease and work-related issues. The emotions surrounding this unpleasant news are likely to engulf work areas as well as almost all aspects of your day-to-day life. Even when most physical symptoms have cleared, unpleasant and troubling invisible symptoms may remain. Problems such as fatigue, numbness, or pain can increase anxiety and interfere with actual job activities. Symptoms such as urinary urgency and frequency may cause embarrassment. Impaired balance can be socially distressing because of its association with consumption of alcohol.

These factors are mentioned only to highlight the emotional turmoil that a person newly diagnosed with MS may experience. This is *not* the frame of mind to have when making critical decisions about work. *Take your time!* Be sure that you have accurate and sufficient information on which to base a decision and that you are emotionally prepared to look objectively at the entire situation—know all your options and their ramifications. Speak with others who have successfully managed MS and/or with a counselor who is experienced in helping people with MS think through the important issues related to employment.

With this background in mind, the following critical points must be emphasized:

• Employment and other productive activities must not be abandoned unnecessarily because of fear and/or misinformation.

• Help is available to assist with work-related decisions and to implement the steps necessary to keep working.

Myths About Multiple Sclerosis

A number of myths or false beliefs make adjustment to MS more difficult. These misconceptions are held not only by a segment of the general public but also by an alarming number of health professionals who do not have extensive experience with MS and/or are unfamiliar with the professional literature. Some of them have a direct impact on the work experience. They include:

• *Stress.* At various points in the history of MS, stress was thought to worsen the disease and escalate the disease process. Scientific studies have examined this issue in detail, and results remain unclear about the role of stress in both the onset and the progression of MS. Advice to quit working, get help to care for children, and curtail volunteer activities is misguided if it is based only on the diagnosis of MS. Specific symptoms may have an impact, but they need to be evaluated individually and carefully because problems may be self-limited or responsive to symptomatic therapy.

- *Activity.* It was formerly believed that physical activity was detrimental to people with MS. The directive was to "take it easy," stop all physical exercise, and rest as much as possible. Bed rest was the primary recommendation for this erratic and unpredictable disease. The major public figure to challenge this notion was Olympic ski medalist Jimmie Heuga, who could not accept a life of inactivity. We now know that Jimmie was right and that activity and exercise are actually beneficial to the well-being of people with MS. It follows that work-related activity should not be curtailed unless dictated by specific, long-standing symptoms that have not responded to therapy.

- *Incapacitation.* Before MS was routinely recognized in its early stages and in mild cases, the common belief was that it would inevitably, and usually quickly, lead to serious disability that would interfere with the ability to perform daily activities, including employment. It is now known that this is not true—most people with MS can often remain active and involved for many years.

Disclosure

The decision to communicate—or not to communicate—the diagnosis of MS in the workplace is complex and important and deserves careful consideration. Disclosure when interviewing for a new job poses different issues from disclosure when you already have an established position.

It is important to be aware of both legal and practical considerations whether you are seeking a new job or maintaining a current one. In the United States, people with disabilities are protected by the Americans with Disabilities Act (ADA), which became law in 1990. The definition of "disability" is complex, but may encompasses MS regardless of whether symptoms are present. This is due to the possible perception of a disability. The employment section of the ADA states that individuals with disabilities who are covered under this law (1) have a mental or physical impairment that substantially limits one or more major life activities; (2) have a history of such an impairment; or (3) are perceived as having such an impairment. A diagnosis of MS carries such a possible preconception since an employer could potentially discriminate based on the association of MS with disability. The ADA prohibits employers from asking about or considering a diagnosis or general limitations in hiring and promotion decisions and only allows questions about ability to perform key components of the job. The ADA does offer the individual the option to request reasonable accommodations in order to perform those essential functions of your job. The challenge is that in order to tap into these protections under law, you would need to disclose that you have a disability and that it does affect one or more major life activities and that the accommodations you are requesting will assist you in effectively and efficiently completing the essential functions of your job. Determining who is the best person to disclose to, the best time to disclose, deciding what to say, and relating disclosure to accommodations are key things to be thinking about. It is important to identify the essential or key elements of your job because nonessential functions may potentially be delegated to or traded with other employees.

In a similar manner, Canadians are protected by the Employment Equity Act (Bill C-64) passed in 1995, which replaces the previous antidiscrimination legislation. This legislation seeks to eliminate employment barriers experienced by women, aboriginals, and visible minorities, as well as people with disabilities. Among the areas of concern that prompted this employment legislation was the severe underrepresentation in the workplace of people with disabilities.

Over time this has begun to change. Both the private and public sectors are covered by Bill C-64. The Act makes use of the Canadian Human Rights Tribunal (called the Employment Equity Review Tribunal when hearing employment equity cases). It also confirms the mandate for Human Resources Development of Canada to conduct research, provide labor market data, and administer programs to recognize outstanding achievement in employment equity. Both appeal procedures and enforcement measures are addressed.

In addition to legal considerations, people with MS are often concerned about health insurance, life insurance, and disability insurance. A prospective or current employee needs to explore policies relative to diagnosis of a chronic disease or occurrence of disability. "Preexisting condition" clauses must be carefully investigated, as well as "caps" (lifetime limits on expenditures for a particular condition or for an individual's total medical expenses) and related categories that potentially limit the availability of medical and health services because of MS or another chronic condition. These factors may or may not be disclosure related, depending on prior documentation of diagnosis and extent of information required for ongoing insurance coverage (see Chapter 8 Financial and Life Planning).

The noninsurance, nonlegal aspects of working with MS often are more difficult to assess and address. Such considerations include anticipated employer and fellow employee support or lack of support, possible growth freeze if limitations are perceived by the employer, and personal emotional investment in efforts to acknowledge or deny issues related to MS. Colleagues, including supervisors, often rally to support a fellow worker with a health problem, In the case of MS, fund-raising teams have sometimes been created to support the individual who has been diagnosed through National MS Society events such as the "Walk" and "Bike Tour." Disclosure relieves the stress of covering up real needs and concerns and mobilizes team spirit and support.

You also need to disclose in order to request necessary accommodations. An accommodation may involve a change in scheduling, a parking space closer to the building entrance, or an office closer to the bathroom. Occasionally, equipment or a structural change such as a ramp may be needed. This is less often the case but usually is accomplished with minimal effort and cost when dealt with directly when the need is first identified.

An employer is required to make arrangements to help an employee perform "essential job functions." These accommodations must be "reasonable" in that they must be affordable and must not impose undue hardship on the employer.

There also are compelling reasons not to disclose: subtle or not so subtle pressure to resign, to accept lesser job responsibilities, or not to apply for promotion or expanded responsibilities. People have reported a "dead-end" feeling if a supervisor has clearly communicated lack of support for further advancement.

Resources

You probably do not need this information now and may never need it. However, you should be aware that such information exists at the time of diagnosis so that you can obtain appropriate assistance at the first sign of difficulty and avoid larger problems altogether. Modest effort early on can prevent serious situations later and support your smooth career development.

Literature is available from the National Multiple Sclerosis Society in the United States (1-800-FIGHT-MS, www.nationalmssociety. org) and the Multiple Sclerosis Society of Canada (416-922-6065, www.mssociety.ca/). Several publications are particularly helpful: *ADA and People with MS* by Cooper, Law and Sarnoff, 2005, which gives details about your protection under law in an easy-to-read style; *The Win-Win Approach to Reasonable Accommodations* by Roessler and Rumrill, 2004, provides a practical guide to obtaining workplace accommodations and covers employment protections under the ADA and disclosure issues; *Should I Work? Information for Employees*, 2003, which gives a general overview of employment issues that might concern people newly diagnosed with MS; *Information for Employers*, 2005, when disclosure has occurred; and *A Place in the Workforce*, 2005, which is a reprint of employment-related articles that originally appeared in *Inside MS*, the magazine of the National MS Society. The articles cover a variety of topics including disclosure, self-employment, and the vocational reabilitaion agency(see Additional Readings).

Each state has a vocational rehabilitation office; the phone number can be obtained through the telephone directory or information assistance, or online at http://www.jan.wvu.edu/sbses/vocrehab. htm. If you look in the blue government pages of the telephone book under "State Government," this agency may be listed under one of the following headings:

- Department of Vocational Rehabilitation

- Department of Rehabilitation

- Department of Human Services

- Department of Social Services

- Department of Social & Rehabitation Services

- Office of Vocational Rehabilitation

Each chapter of the National MS Society has a designated person who can address common employment issues. This "employment advisor" may be a trained chapter staff or volunteer in the community who is familiar with employment concerns of people with MS. This person will be able to address your questions and refer you to other employment resources and agencies.

In 2005, the National MS Society created the Career Crossroads: Employment and MS program. This program comprises a workbook and video/DVD that addresses common employment issues including disclosure, accommodation strategies, legal rights and responsibilities (ADA, FMLA), insurance issues (HIPAA, COBRA), and resources. Chapters may offer this training periodically, and the format may vary from chapter-to-chapter.

Some important resources include:

- Job Accommodation Network (JAN), 1-800-526-7234, www.jan. wvu.edu

- JAN ADA Information Line, 1-800-ADA-WORK (1-800-232-9675

- ADA&IT Technical Assistance Centers, 1-800-949-4232, www.adata.org

- Equal Employment Opportunity Commission (EEOC), 1-800-669-4000, 1-800669-6820 (TDD), www.eeoc.gov

- U.S, Department of Justice ADA Information Line, 1-800-514-0301, www.ada.gov

The U.S. and Canadian MS Societies have a general program for people recently diagnosed with MS called Knowledge is Power, which can be accessed by calling 1-800-FIGHT-MS in the United States (www.nationalmssociety.org) and 416-922-6065 in Canada (www.mssociety.ca/). Society chapters also have periodic educational programs for people recently diagnosed with MS and their families and include issues relative to employment.

8

||||||||||||||||||||||||||||||||||||||||||||||||||||||||||||||||||||||||||||||||||||||||||||||||||||||||||||||

*Financial and Life Planning**

One part of dealing with multiple sclerosis (MS) is managing your money and planning wisely for the future. Just as your MS symptoms are not exactly like someone else's symptoms, your financial situation also is unique. Now more than ever, you will need to take a clear look at your income, assets, debts, benefits, and other resources.

At first glance, getting a good handle on your finances may seem overwhelming. If you give yourself some time and have a little patience, however, you can accomplish this step.

> *When I was first diagnosed with MS, I asked "Am I going to die?" The doctor said that, yes, someday I would die–but not from MS. That was more than 25 years ago. Since then, I've had my ups and downs, but I'm still around, I still love life, and I've always managed to find a way to pay for the things I need.*
>
> —Leslie, diagnosed in 1980

---

*Modified with permission from *Adapting: Financial Planning for a Life with Multiple Sclerosis* produced by the National Endowment for Financial Education.

Getting Organized

An important first step is to gather the following materials. It is helpful to make copies and put them in labeled file folders in one location that you can get to easily.

- Birth certificate

- Checking and savings account information

- Durable power of attorney document

- Employee benefits information

- Insurance policies (life, health, disability, and long-term care)

- Investment account information

- Loans, including credit card statements

- Marriage certificate

- Military records

- Mortgage/deed of trust

- Social Security card

- Tax returns

- Titles (e.g., auto, house)

- Will

Professional Advisors

It is important to include the names and contact information of your professional advisors with your financial file folders.

	ADVISOR'S NAME	PHONE NUMBER
Accountant/tax preparer		
Financial planner		
Insurance agent		
Lawyer		
Other		

Taking a Financial Inventory

Review your MS symptoms to see if any of them may lead to additional expenses. For example, you may need to pay for regular massages to lessen muscle stiffness, or buy an air conditioner to keep your home cool because of sensitivity to heat. The spending plan worksheets, found on pages 137–139 also can help you estimate your monthly income and expenses.

Next, write down an estimated value of everything you own and the dollar amount of your debts. You'll want this information as you plan for future expenses or apply for any benefits that are based on financial need. As you do this estimate, take into consideration the Internal Revenue Service's definitions of value (go to www.irs.gov) and consider obtaining a professional appraisal of valuable assets, such as your home, artwork, jewelry, or other collectibles. Your accountant or other financial advisor can guide you.

Using a Health-Expense Spreadsheet

Another step you or a loved one can take is to create a health-expense spreadsheet (sample on page 130). The spreadsheet should list items such as:

- Dates of doctor visits, hospital stays, or other treatments

- Charges for medical services, prescriptions, and medical supplies

- Portions of expenses covered by a health-care plan

- Amounts and dates that you paid for health-care services and any remaining balances

- Dates any deductibles were met, if applicable

Software programs can help you create a spreadsheet and will even do the math for you. If you do not own a computer, you can create a spreadsheet in a notebook or use the one provided on page 130. Remember to keep copies of your supporting paperwork: doctor bills, health insurance statements, canceled checks, and bank statements in labeled file folders.

Realize that mistakes can happen when medical claims are processed. Even though these mistakes usually are unintentional, they can be costly. Check with your health-care plan to see if it will share savings resulting from any errors you find in medical bills. Take careful notes while in the hospital or receiving treatment, and check the bill against your notes.

If you find possible billing errors, first try to resolve them with the doctor's or hospital's billing office. Next, get in touch with your health insurance company.

If the matter remains unresolved, contact your state's consumer protection office or insurance regulatory agency to file a complaint. Look in the blue pages of the phone book.

Reviewing Your Health-Care Plan

As soon as possible, review your health-care plan, so you will know what the plan will cover, what is excluded, and what your out-of-pocket expenses may be. Having this information will help you plan for anticipated medical expenses and strengthen an appeal on a claim if you believe it was denied incorrectly.

Health-care plans can be difficult to read and understand, but there are people who can help you. Check the back of your health-care card for

Health-Expense Spreadsheet

DATE OF SERVICE/ MEDICAL PURCHASE	CHARGES	AMOUNT/ DATE PAID BY HEALTH- CARE PLAN*	AMOUNT/ DATE PAID BY ME	DATE DEDUCTIBLE AND/OR COINSURANCE MET	DATE OUT-OF- POCKET LIMIT REACHED

phone numbers to call for information about your plan. If your health-care plan is provided through an employer, someone in the employee benefits department may be able to answer your questions.

When reviewing your plan, determine if it is a major-medical plan or a managed-care plan, such as a health maintenance organization (HMO), preferred provider organization (PPO), or point-of-service plan (POS). Pay particular attention to information about copayments, coinsurance, deductibles, preexisting condition exclusion periods, lifetime maximums, and prescription drugs. These topics are discussed in the following sections.

Copayment

Most managed-care plans require you to pay a small amount, called the copayment or copay, each time you visit a health-care provider within the plan's network. The amount of the copay may change annually. If your plan also has a deductible, the copay will not count toward it. Major-medical plans and some major medical-type benefits under managed-care plans do not have a copay.

Deductible

A deductible is the amount you must pay each year before a major-medical plan pays any expenses. For example, if your health-care plan has a $500 deductible, you must pay the first $500 of covered medical costs before the plan begins to kick in. (If the treatment is not covered by the plan, the cost for that treatment will not count toward the deductible.) Managed-care plans, such as a PPO, HMO, or POS, may have a deductible if they permit care from out-of-network providers. Review your plan to determine which provisions apply to the provider you want to use.

Coinsurance

Coinsurance is the portion of a health-care expense that you pay in addition to the deductible (when these provisions are part of your plan). A typical coinsurance provision says that after the deductible is paid, the health-care plan pays 80 percent of covered charges for a treatment. You pay the other 20 percent. The percentage is your coinsurance amount. Plans very as to the amount they expect you to pay.

Most plans have a "stop-loss," "breakpoint," or "out-of-pocket" limit. This is the maximum amount you will have to pay per person, or per family, each year. For example, an insurance company may have a stop-loss of $5,000. After you have paid $5,000 in deductible and coinsurance payments, the insurance company will pay 100 percent of covered expenses for the rest of the year. Check your plan for details.

Covered Expenses

Regardless of the amount charged by a provider, a plan will only cover certain treatments for certain amounts. Make sure you know what your plan considers a "covered expense," and if your health-care provider will accept the plan's payment or will bill you for any amounts not covered by the plan.

Preexisting Condition Exclusion Period

A preexisting condition is a medical problem you had before you joined a health-care plan. With a preexisting condition, you may have to wait a period of time before the plan will cover that medical condition. This length of time could be 3 months, 6 months, or 1 year. As a rule, a group health plan cannot make you wait more than 1 year unless you did not enroll in the plan when first offered, in which case the waiting period may be as long as 18 months.

Under the Health Insurance Portability and Accountability Act (HIPAA) of 1996, you will not have to meet a preexisting condition exclusion period under a new plan if:

- You have had medical coverage for 18 months before changing to a new plan.

- You already have met a preexisting condition exclusion period under a previous plan.

- You have not been without health-care coverage for more than 62 days in the last 12 months.

Lifetime Maximums

Health-care plans usually limit how much they will pay for health care through a "lifetime maximum benefit." When the limit is reached, the health-care plan no longer pays for medical care. There also may be a limit for a single illness, injury, or condition, or an annual limit on certain medical services or equipment.

Prescription Drugs

Drugs for MS can be expensive. For example, the major drugs approved by the Food and Drug Administration (FDA) for relapsing-remitting MS can cost between $10,000 and $14,000 a year. Plus, you likely will require other medications to manage symptoms. Even if your health-care plan offers prescription drug coverage, you may have to pay part of the cost of these medications, so it is important to plan for this expense.

Start by finding out whether the medications you need are covered by your health-care plan. This information is available in the plan's "formulary," which is a list of drugs the plan will cover. Many health-care plans cover the drugs that have been shown to modify the course of MS.

If you are having difficulty paying for your medications, consider the following options:

- The companies that manufacture the major disease-modifying drugs may offer prescription drug assistance programs. Each program has its own qualifications. Begin by reading *Comparing the Disease-Modifying Drugs*, published by the National Multiple Sclerosis Society (www.nationalmssociety.org).

- Information about other prescription drug assistance programs for people with limited resources can be found at www.phrma.org. Several states also have prescription drug assistance programs.

- Talk to your doctor about prescribing a less expensive drug or helping you apply for a prescription drug assistance program.

- Shop for the best price and the best pharmacy. Compare local prices with mail order or online pharmacies, including delivery charges. If you decide to use a mail order or online pharmacy, choose one that requires a written prescription from your doctor. Be careful about using foreign pharmacies because of the importance of ensuring that the product you order is genuine, of the right strength, and uncontaminated.

- Order a copy of *Free and Low Cost Prescription Drugs*. This 48-page booklet from the nonprofit Cost Containment Research Institute lists nearly 1,200 brand-name drugs available from drug companies at a large discount for those who qualify. The booklet costs about $5. For ordering information, visit the Institute's Web site at www.institutedc.org.

- If you are a veteran, you may qualify for Department of Veterans Affairs (VA) health benefits, which include prescription drugs. You must enroll to receive benefits.

Family and Medical Leave Act

The Family and Medical Leave Act (FMLA) of 1993 requires employers with 50 or more workers, and all public/government employers, to provide up to 12 weeks of unpaid leave a year to eligible employees coping with certain family or medical situations. You can take the leave in small increments or all at once to care for yourself or an immediate family member, with the guarantee that you can keep your job and your health-care benefits. Generally, the employer may decide whether FMLA time can be taken in installments.

To be eligible for FMLA leave, an employee must:

- Work for an employer that is covered by FMLA

- Have worked at the company for a total of 12 months

- Have worked at least 1,250 hours during the past 12 months

Employers may require employees to provide medical certification supporting the need for a leave due to a serious health condition affecting the employee or an immediate family member. In addition, when intermittent leave is needed for medical treatment, the employee must try to schedule the treatment so as not to unduly disrupt the employer's business.

Short-Term Disability Insurance

You may have disability insurance through your employer or on your own. The insurance might pay you a benefit if you experience either a short-term or a long-term disability that prevents you from working.

Keep in mind that even though an exacerbation is temporary, it can be disabling. Short-term disability insurance can help you through these times. With short-term disability insurance, which usually is available only through an employer, you can qualify for benefits within a few days or weeks of becoming disabled. The benefits can stop after a varied number of months, depending on the policy. Typically, you will be paid about 40 to 60 percent of your wages. You must report the benefit as taxable income if the employer paid the premiums for the insurance.

Job Changes and Health Care

One of the most important job benefits an employer can offer is a health-care plan. Because MS is a lifelong condition, carefully consider the heath benefits provided by an employer before accepting a position. Or, if you currently work for a company that does not offer a health-care plan, you may want to look for a new job that has health-care benefits.

In addition to COBRA, the Health Insurance Portability and Accountability Act of 1996 (HIPAA), also known as the Kennedy-Kassenbaum Act, provides protection to individuals with a preexisting condition when moving to a new health plan. HIPAA limits exclusions for preexisting conditions and prohibits discrimination against employees and dependents based on their health status. This law guarantees that most workers with preexisting conditions can move from their former group health plan to their new employees plan without a break in coverage. For more information on HIPAA, go to www.dol.gov/pwba.

Don't ask to see the benefits package during the first interview, but when offered a job, ask to review the package before giving an answer. When reviewing the health-care portion of the employer's benefits package, pay particular attention to the:

- Waiting period

- Preexisting condition exclusion period

- Plan benefits and your costs

Taking Control of Finances

Developing a Spending Plan

The best way to know how much money you need to live on every month is to make a spending plan. Consider making several copies of

STEP 1: IDENTIFY YOUR INCOME

MONTHLY INCOME WORKSHEET	
SOURCES	PER MONTH ($)
After-tax wages	
Tips or bonuses	
Child support	
Alimony/maintenance payment(s)	
Unemployment compensation	
Social Security or Supplemental Security Income	
Retirement plan(s)	
Private disability insurance payments	
VA benefits	
Public assistance	
Food stamps	
Interest/investment income	
Other	
Total Income:	

STEP 2: LIST EXPENSES

MONTHLY INCOME WORKSHEET	
SOURCES	PER MONTH ($)
Mortgage or rent	
Utilities (heat, electricity, and water)	
Telephone, cellphone, Internet provider	
Groceries	
Transportation (bus fare, car payment, gas, repairs)	
Insurance (cost per month for car, home, health, and life insurance	
Housekeeper/gardener, etc.	
Prescription drugs, medical supplies, and equipment	
Treatments or therapies (massage, exercise classes, alternative treatments, supplements, etc.)	
Doctor/dentist bills	
Home adaptations or improvements	
Clothing/uniforms	
Child care/child support payments	
Alimony/maintenance payments	
Loan/credit care payments	
Entertainment (movies, eating out, etc.)	
Miscellaneous (e.g.,classes, gifts, vacations, pet care)	
Donations	
Taxes	
Savings/retirement plan contributions*	
Other	
Total Expenses:	

*Think of saving money as a regular monthly expense. That way, you will be more likely to save.

STEP 3: COMPARE INCOME AND EXPENSES

Write down your total monthly income (from Step 1).	$
Write down your total monthly expenses (from Step 2).	$
Subtract expenses from income and list amount here.	$

the spending plan worksheets so you can use them throughout the year, or whenever your financial situation changes.

Looking at Investments

You may have money in a 401(K) or other retirement plan, or have other investments. It is a good idea to periodically review where your money is invested. The challenge is to find the right balance between the financial risk you can tolerate and the need for your money to grow.

If you currently are putting money into an employer-provided retirement plan, try to continue doing so. This is one of the best ways to save for your future—and you get special tax breaks. In addition, employers often match all or part of the money you save in the plan. Put at least enough money into the retirement plan to qualify for matching dollars from your employer.

Hiring a Financial Professional

If you decide to hire a financial planner to review your finances, ask the MS Society to refer you to professionals who have worked with people diagnosed with MS. The National MS Society in the United States has developed a partnership with the Society of Financial Professionals called the Financial Education Partners which will provide volunteer professionals to meet one-on-one with people with MS. Be sure to call the Society at 1-800- FIGHT MS about this opportunity. In addition, the following organizations can provide names of financial planners near you:

- American Institute of Certified Public Accountants, Personal Financial Planning Division, www.cpapfs.org

- Financial Planning Association, www.fpanet.org

- National Association of Personal Financial Advisors, www.napfa.org

- Society of Financial Service Professionals, www.financialpro.org

Setting Aside Money for Unexpected Expenses

Many financial experts advise putting aside enough money to cover your bills for 3 to 6 months. This money can help if you lose your job or face other unexpected costs. Because you are dealing with a chronic disease, try to save enough money to cover 6 months of expenses.

The money you set aside for unexpected events should be placed in an account that you can get to easily. Consider the following options:

- **Savings account.** Savings accounts are easy to open and offer quick access to your money. While they pay only a small amount of interest, savings accounts at banks, savings and loans, and credits unions are safe investments.

- **Money market account.** You often need $1,000 to $10,000 to open a money market account. You may earn more interest on this type of account than with a savings account, but you may have limited access to it. In addition, depending on where you open a money market account, it may not be insured by the federal government. Be sure to ask.

- **Roth IRA.** Even though IRA stands for Individual Retirement Account, you can use a Roth IRA as a way to set money aside for emergencies. Unlike a regular IRA, you can withdraw the after-tax money you put into a Roth IRA without paying a penalty or taxes. However, generally you *cannot* withdraw any interest the account earns until age 59½ without paying a penalty. You are not taxed on any of the money you withdraw from a Roth IRA provided that you withdraw the money after age 59½, and the Roth IRA has been in existence for at least 5 years. However, if you become disabled, and distributions are made because of your disability, you do not have to meet the age 59½ rule for distributions of earnings to be income tax free.

To learn more about saving, investing, and personal finance, ask your librarian to recommend several good books. Or, take a look at the following Web sites: Alliance for Investor Education, www.investoreducation.org; American Savings Education Council, www.asec.org; Investment Company Institute, www.ici.org; or National Endowment for Financial Education, www.nefe.org.

9

||||||||||||||||||||||||||||||||||||||||||||||||||||||||||||||||||||||||||||||||||||||||||||||||||||||||||||||||||||||

Research in Multiple Sclerosis: The Search for Answers and the Link to Treatments

Research in multiple sclerosis (MS) can help uncover fundamental knowledge of the disease's cause, its relationship to other diseases, and to its course. This information is essential for developing safe and effective therapies that are as specific for MS as possible. Indeed, it is hard to conceive of treatments, prevention, or a cure for MS ever happening without a vigorous and critical international research effort.

MS research began in the mid-1800s as simple descriptive studies that examined the symptoms of the disease and its effect on nervous system tissue. It has evolved now, more than 150 years later, into a specialty area of basic and clinical research that incorporates virtually every discipline of modern biotechnology, ranging from the most up-to-date molecular laboratory techniques to studies of population, socioeconomics, and psychology and to the testing of new therapies for their safety and efficacy.

Scientific research is a specialized discipline. Scientists are trained not only in their area of specialty research but also in the discipline of scientific inquiry. Simple "observation" is a form of scientific inquiry that is most useful in initial studies. The observation of biologic processes and how they may change, as in disease, can help generate important new theories about the disease cause and treatment, which can then be tested in more rigorous fashion.

Scientific research is driven by specific theories or hypotheses using controlled laboratory or clinical techniques that have the greatest likelihood of providing meaningful answers. A *hypothesis* is a tentative assumption, usually developed through early observational study that can be proved or disproved in the course of investigation.

Most modern MS research is related to four major hypotheses about the disease and its cause (see Chapter 2): (1) it is an auto-immune disease; (2) it occurs in genetically susceptible individuals; (3) it is triggered by some infectious or environmental factor; and (4) it results in immune system–mediated inflammation and loss of the white matter (myelin) and underlying nerve fibers of the brain and spinal cord, bringing neurologic symptoms and the associated socioeconomic problems long recognized to occur with MS.

Research in Immunology—Uncovering the Root of the Disease

While MS is recognized as a disease of the brain, spinal cord, and optic nerves (the central nervous system [CNS]), it is widely believed that the characteristic neurologic signs and symptoms of MS are caused by an immune system disorder that causes damage to CNS tissue and disrupts the normal activity of the part of the CNS controlling movement, sensory perception, thinking, and emotional functioning.

Our body's immune system is highly complex and includes lymphocytes (T cells), antibodies, a host of regulatory substances that circulate in the blood called *cytokines* and *chemokines*, and many other key players. Normal immune function protects the body from injury and disease caused by infectious agents—such as bacteria, viruses, and parasites—by mounting an attack against the "invaders" and clearing them from the body. Because our immune systems and our tissues and organs are all part and parcel of ourselves, each individual's body tissues are usually protected and not subject to attack by his or her own immune system. This "self-protection" is rooted in the identical genetic make-up of each person's immune system and other organs and tissues: The identical genetic background signals that the tissues are a normal part of the body and should not be considered to be foreign invaders.

Sometimes, however, this innate protection goes awry and a person's own immune system begins to attack his or her own body tissues and organs as though they were foreign. Most scientists believe that this is the root cause of MS: The disease is the result of an abnormality in which a person's own immune system fails to distinguish foreign invaders (like viruses and bacteria) from normal tissues in the body. As a consequence, the immune system attacks apparently normal body tissues as well as foreign invaders, resulting in inflammation and tissue damage that is often permanent. This "self-attack" of the immune system against a person's own body tissues is termed *autoimmunity.*

Efforts to understand autoimmunity are the largest area of research in MS worldwide. Immunologic research related to MS has progressed over the years from identifying immune cells in the nervous system, where they do not normally belong, to understanding how immune system components are regulated and become dysfunctional in autoimmune disease. Understanding immune function in the disease has helped to reveal important aspects of its cause and has resulted in virtually all of the innovative new therapies for controlling MS disease course that are available today. We are now in a position to marshal this growing body of vital information about immune system function and dysfunction into the development of a new generation of potential therapies for MS.

Studies have been undertaken in healthy individuals to better understand normal immune system functioning in individuals with MS to learn what goes wrong in the disease; and in individuals with other autoimmune diseases, such as rheumatoid arthritis and juvenile-onset diabetes,to understand what these disorders can tell us more generally about immune system abnormalities and autoimmunity in particular.

In addition to human studies, immunologic research in MS has been greatly aided by work with the laboratory animal model disease *experimental allergic (or autoimmune) encephalomyelitis* (EAE), a laboratory-induced autoimmune disease of the brain and spinal cord in rats, mice, guinea pigs, and nonhuman primates that has many characteristics in common with MS. Studies of animal models for MS and related animal model diseases for other human autoimmune disorders have greatly facilitated our understanding of basic immune system function and what goes wrong in autoimmune diseases. While in no case are these animal disorders exactly like MS (for instance, they are all laboratory-induced diseases, while MS in humans is, as far as we know it, a spontaneous disease) they are a practical, relatively rapid way to obtain answers to difficult questions and to generate hypotheses that can be tested in future humans studies.

Because MS involves the immune system, for several decades physicians have used powerful drugs that suppress immune function by decreasing the growth and proliferation of immune cells. Many such therapies that have been tested for MS—drugs such as cyclophosphamide and azathioprine and procedures such as total body or total lymphoid irradiation—have global or widespread immunosuppressive effects, potentially leaving a treated patient open to a variety of infections and complications. This complication has made these therapies of questionable value in terms of cost versus benefit. Even while recognizing that some of these agents might be able to help control the disease process, the risks of using them in terms of future problems, such as malignancies, has limited their acceptance and use. However, at least one such agent, mitoxantrone (sold as Novantrone®), has found regulatory and clinical acceptance for "worsening MS," especially in patients who have not responded well to other therapies. And other such global immunosuppressive agents are currently under investigation in human clinical trials.

However, given the potential risk of global immunosuppressive agents, the need for more specific immune therapy approaches that may not have global immunosuppressive risks has been recognized for many years. To this end, pinpointing the immune problems more exactly in MS has long been a goal, with the belief that such information could lead to highly specific therapies aimed at those immune system components involved in the disease, while leaving the rest of the immune system intact and functioning.

As a consequence, the search to understand the specific immune responses involved in MS has been an important focus of research in recent years. This includes exploring what makes an immune system that is normally directed against outside invaders become misdirected against normal body tissues (mistaking "self" tissue for "foreign" invaders); searching for the actual target of immune responses in the brain and spinal cord (the "antigen" that triggers immune attack and that could be the target of specific therapies); and determining the nature of T cells and antibodies that are primed to attack this target.

Another promising avenue of immunologic research has sought to understand how and why immune system cells move from the blood stream into the CNS. This phenomenon, called trafficking, may be one of the most important aspects of immune system problems in MS. Ordinarily, activated immune cells that could cause damage in the CNS are prevented from moving from the blood (where they normally circulate throughout the body to do protective immune surveillance) to the nervous system, where they can do damage. In MS, the blood-brain barrier (BBB) that keeps activated immune cells in the blood is breached and the potentially damaging cells enter the nervous system. Why is the BBB breached in MS? How can the resulting movement of cells into the nervous system be stopped? Within recent years, a sufficient body of information has accumulated that has allowed the development of specific therapies that can block the BBB breach and reduce or prevent immune cell trafficking in MS. One such agent, a monoclonal antibody, natalizumab (marketed as Tysabri®) has been shown to be very successful in reducing the rate of MS relapses and in slowing progression of disability and in 2006 won regulatory approval from the U.S. Food and Drug Administration (FDA) for use in relapsing forms of the disease; even in the face of significant potential toxicity of the agent that will likely limit its widespread use. Continuing work in the area of immune cell trafficking is essential if we are to complete the biologic picture of MS and develop additional treatments that safely and effectively reduce or prevent such trafficking.

Not all hypotheses and studies are successful in MS immunologic research (or in any other branch of research). For example, in the late 1980s, with considerable background information on immune responses in EAE in mice, scientists reported evidence that there were relatively few potential disease-causing brain antigens—targets of the disease process—in myelin insulation tissue surrounding nerve fibers. They also reported that they were able to identify T cells specific for those antigens and, they believed, specifically tied to the MS disease process. With this information, a number of scientists and pharmaceutical companies began to design specifically engineered antibodies (immune system proteins produced in the laboratory that have the ability to target and neutralize specific proteins) and synthetic peptides (parts of proteins) aimed at preventing immune system attack against the target antigens in myelin in the CNS. In the animal model for MS, EAE, disease could be prevented entirely with such techniques, and improvement was seen when disease was already present before treatment using such interventions.

This work generated enormous excitement and many hypotheses for treating MS in humans. However, the immune response against myelin in humans turned out to be much more complicated than in the laboratory animal model disease. There are, in fact, multiple myelin antigens involved in immune system responses in humans and likely in MS as a consequence, and different people may have different antigenic responses. And over time, there tends to be a shifting in immune responses, so the target of the immune response in myelin may change in the course of disease in a given individual. This means that specific T-cell treatments aimed at taking advantage of the originally proposed "restricted" immune responses in MS are not likely to be effective for a wide spectrum of patients with MS, and treatments effective at one time in the disease may not continue to be effective.

One relatively new focus in immunologic research in MS has been on chemical messengers of the immune system called *cytokines* and *chemokines*. Cytokines and chemokines are produced by immune and other cells that regulate immune system activity. Many scientists believe that cytokines may be important "final pathways" involved in all immune responses—some cytokines encourage inflammation, which can be damaging in MS, and others suppress inflammation, which may be protective in MS. By manipulating cytokine activity so that proinflammatory responses are suppressed and anti-inflammatory responses are encouraged, it may not be necessary to understand specific immune cell responses in MS to combat the disease. And a second group of immune messengers, chemokines, send important information signals throughout the body, helping to direct immune responses where they need to be most active. Controlling these chemical messengers may provide a kind of relatively nonspecific treatment for MS.

Early studies showed that some cytokines and chemokines may make EAE and MS worse and others may make the diseases better. Interferons, which are one type of cytokine, are an example of this dichotomy: Interferon beta has been shown to be anti-inflammatory and has been beneficial for treating MS, while there is evidence that interferon gamma may make the disease worse, at least at certain stages of the disease. Thus, enhancing the activity of interferons beta might be an effective treatment; suppressing gamma interferons at certain states of the disease might be successful as well. In fact, no fewer than three approved therapies for MS provide interferon beta by injection.

Work underway continues to gain a better understanding of the cytokine "networks" and chemokine signaling pathways that are involved in MS and to learn how to block "bad" cytokines and chemokines and enhance the effects of "good" ones—all toward the ultimate goal of providing safe and effective disease treatments. Much of our fundamental understanding of such immune system information networks comes, again, from laboratory animal model diseases and from research in other immune-mediated human diseases.

Much about immunology and autoimmunity, including the actions of cytokines and chemokines, is shared among different diseases which are thought to be autoimmune in origin. However, even if such complex immune networks are understood in a different disease, the outcomes are not always predictable in MS. For example, an important cytokine called tumor necrosis factor alpha (TNFα) was found to be involved in nervous system tissue damage in animal models of MS and believed to be functioning abnormally in MS itself. Blocking the action of TNFα in EAE prevented or improved disease. A similar phenomenon was seen in animal models of rheumatoid arthritis, which resulted in successful clinical trials for an agent that blocks TNFα in that disease, which is now available to treat arthritis patients. However, surprisingly, in preliminary clinical studies in humans with MS, use of such TNFα blockers caused an *increase* in MS-related lesions in the brain, which is a clear indication that this approach could not be easily used in MS and might, in fact, be harmful. So, as informative as animal and other disease research may be for MS, it is impossible to predict MS-specific results. This is why careful, stepwise research needs to be conducted. But this TNFα setback does not negate the potential value of controlling cytokine activity in MS. Another cytokine, called interleukin-2 (IL-2), can foster harmful inflammatory activity in the brain in animal models and in MS, and a monoclonal antibody that can block the activity of IL-2, successful in treatment of EAE, is now in clinical testing in MS.

While most work in MS immunology has focused on the T-cell response, cytokines and chemokines, antibodies produced by B cells are increasingly believed to be important in MS pathology as well.

Antibodies have been found in MS lesions in the brain and have been linked to disease pathology in certain forms of EAE and human MS. These studies have been essential in pointing out a new direction not only in fundamental research in MS but also in developing concepts for treatment: Certain kinds of immune therapies that can "improve" T-cell–mediated disease can actually make antibody-mediated disease worse and vice versa. Therefore, a better understanding of the relative roles of T cells and antibodies in disease pathology in different individuals, and perhaps at different stages of disease in the same individual, has important treatment implications and the potential to unveil key aspects of the underlying disease phenomenon. The recent focus on antibodies as an important part of the MS pathology has led to attempts to control antibody responses using agents that specifically block the immune B cells that produce them. Clinical trials of B-cell blockers, following upon years of more fundamental research, are underway in both relapsing and primary progressive forms of MS.

An important adjunct to immunologic research is the role of hormones in MS. It is well known that MS is two to three times as common in women as in men; a gender bias that is seen in many diseases considered to be autoimmune in nature. And it is well known that pregnant women with MS tend to have stabilization or improvement of their disease in the second and third trimesters of pregnancy, when estrogen levels are high, only to experience a higher risk for a disease exacerbation in the first several months after delivery, when estrogen levels drop. Changes in estrogen levels during pregnancy are thought to help regulate immune function: The immune system needs to be suppressed in pregnancy to prevent a "rejection" of the fetus, which is recognized as being foreign by the mother's immune system. (This is because the fetal genetic make-up, a combination of the genes of the mother and the father, is fundamentally incompatible with the mother's immune system genetics, and thus immune responses may be mounted against the fetus).

Therefore, hormone regulation of immune responses in MS has been an important area of MS research in recent years. Estrogen, a female sex hormone, actually can improve EAE, the animal model of MS; testosterone, a male sex hormone, can make the disease worse. Would hormone levels also help control MS in humans by regulating immune function? This key new aspect of our understanding of MS immunology has led to promising clinical trials in both women and men with MS designed to determine whether the use of estrogen or testosterone can help mediate disease.

Genetic Research—Links to Susceptibility, Course, and Causation

Research on the genetic basis of MS has resulted in vast amounts of new information in a decade and a half. Basic population studies tell us that specific groups of people in the world may be protected from MS and others may be more susceptible (see Chapter 2). Moving beyond population studies, genetics research has become highly "molecular" in nature as scientists race to uncover genetic factors that underlie the disease and may help determine who is susceptible to developing MS. The worldwide effort to reveal the total human genetic code—completed at the end of 2000—has helped us understand the genetic code that defines humans and was the first step in unraveling the complexities of diseases with genetic components. Whole genomic screens in MS, while they have not defined the genetic basis of the disease, have supported hypotheses about its autoimmune nature. Genomic screen studies have now led to a focus on analysis of genetic haplotypes—blocks of genes that tend to be inherited together and which may be used for easier analysis of genetic factors in diseases like MS.

The possibility of specific gene therapies is no longer the stuff of science fiction, even though its application to human disease is far from straightforward today. In humans in whom this has been tried, for instance, in metabolic diseases and more recently in muscular dystrophy, the safety and efficacy of such approaches has been far from certain, and there are significant ethical and governmental restraints on gene therapy studies in humans. For gene therapy to become a potential treatment in a disease like MS, we need to understand completely the genetic factors that underlie the disease and devise ways to "correct" any defects that may be present. We are a long way from this goal and, given the nature of the disease, it may not be possible to achieve it at all.

A more immediate consequence of genetic research in MS may be the development of techniques to more readily determine susceptibility to MS in the general population and in families in which the disease already occurs. Genetic factors may even one day provide some clues to the prognosis for any individual with the disease, helping to predict the type of MS that a person will have and even its severity.

An interesting consequence of genetics research has been a boost to the belief that MS is autoimmune in nature. Immune function is under strict genetic control, and the genes of people with MS that control immune function are in some ways different from the immune system genes of healthy individuals. Among these are genes involved in helping the immune system determine which body tissues are its own ("self") and which substances are foreign—a bacterium or virus or even a transplanted liver or kidney from a genetically different donor. This ability to distinguish between self and foreign allows the immune system to mount an effective response against foreign substances but not against tissues or cells that are part of its own body. Genes controlling this recognition process are called human leukocyte antigens (HLA genes), histocompatibility genes, or major histocompatibility genes (MHC genes). Based on both early population studies in which HLA typing was done on blood samples and more recent results from highly molecular state of the art whole genome screens of individuals with MS in the United States, Canada, and the United Kingdom, the HLA genes are, to date, the strongest link that we have to an MS genetic factor.

Thus, at their most basic level, genetic studies are helping us to know more about the immune nature of the disease, how much of the disease susceptibility may be related to genetic problems in immune system function, and how much of it may be related to other nonimmunologic factors or even to environmental or infectious factors.

Infectious Disease Research—Clues to Triggers, Causes, and Possibly Treatments

Genes and the immune system are clearly involved with MS, but what event actually triggers the development of MS in people who are susceptible? That is where infectious disease research plays a role. Over the decades, some rare infectious agents have been proposed to be linked to MS, but more often, very common viruses and bacteria—agents that infect the majority of individuals in the population whether or not they have MS—have been the focus of attention.

Viral infections can cause human diseases with characteristics similar to those of MS, and certain viral diseases in laboratory animals also result in myelin damage like that seen in MS. For decades there has been very clear evidence that some viral infections, particularly upper respiratory tract viral infections, may set off acute exacerbations of MS in individuals who already have the disease. These observations, coupled with the rather unusual geographic spread of MS (more common in temperate regions; rare in tropical regions), have generated years of scientific hypotheses concerning infectious agents and MS.

Researchers have hunted for a specific identifiable virus related to MS, with the hope that this will result in a relatively simple explanation for the disease, and also with the hope that combating such a virus with a specific vaccination will result in a safe and effective preventative (as was the case in the control of poliomyelitis beginning in the 1950s) or a specific virus-focused disease treatment. However, the search for *the* MS virus has been unfruitful. Several dozen common and uncommon viruses have been postulated to be specifically related to MS based on either epidemiologic studies, the presence of higher levels of antibodies against a given virus in individuals with MS, or, more recently, evidence from very sophisticated polymerase chain reaction

(PCR) analysis that can detect the "footprint" of a viral protein in body fluids and tissues even if the virus has been long eliminated by the immune system.

In virtually every case of such claims, however, follow-up studies that are needed to confirm a relationship to MS (confirmation of results is an essential part of the scientific process!) have been unsuccessful. Most such claims have been a result of inadequate experimental sampling or laboratory contamination. Nonetheless, there remains the possibility that specific infections may be related to MS, and virologists who focus on this disease are at the forefront of ongoing searches.

In recent years, most of the focus has been on viruses that are very common in the general population—not necessarily isolated only in individuals with MS—such as human herpesvirus 6 (HHV6), which causes roseola in infants, and Epstein-Barr virus (EBV), which is known as the cause of infectious mononucleosis. Virtually everyone in the population has been exposed to these viruses, but not everyone has MS! But both epidemiologic and biologic studies have suggested a strong association between HHV6 infection and MS and between EBV infection, mononucleosis in childhood or adolescence and later development of MS. These observations and associations have generated many hypotheses that are being actively explored, yet a causative relationship for either with MS has not yet been proven. A common bacterial infection has similarly been linked to MS. *Chlamydia pneumoniae*, the cause of "walking pneumonia," is an infectious agent to which most humans have been exposed. Reports have claimed an association with this bacterium in individuals with MS and have shown its presence in MS tissues. But many years of follow-up research have raised skepticism about the original reports, and a causal relationship between this bacterium and MS has not been proven.

How can common infectious agents be involved with MS when relatively few humans have the disease? Are these false leads and not really causes of MS? Are such agents simply associated with MS or are they "cofactors" that are required, but not in themselves sufficient, to cause the disease? If so, what else might be required for the disease to appear? This is where *genetic susceptibility* may have its impact: While a common infectious agent may be a trigger for MS, perhaps the disease will only occur in people who carry a genetic susceptibility to it. Is it possible that both—a triggering agent and the "right" genetic background—are required and neither alone is sufficient for MS to develop?

This may be the case, but many investigators believe it is likely that no specific virus, bacterium, or other infectious agent will be found to be a cause of MS. Rather, they are concentrating on research that explores how a susceptible person's immune system reacts to a variety of viral or other infections, or how immune function is tied to hormonal and other factors that might explain the initiation of the MS process. Studies from the mid-1990s through the current time, largely in laboratory animals, have helped to explain how an immune system that has lost its ability to distinguish self from nonself tissue can be tricked by certain infectious agents into mounting an attack against a person's own myelin. The "trick" might be a very close similarity of molecular structure between some viruses, bacteria, and myelin itself—called molecular mimicry to reflect the similarity of molecular structure between some parts of myelin and some infectious agents. An effective and natural immune response mounted against a common infectious agent might result in a damaging cross-reaction with myelin itself if the molecular structure of the infectious agent mimics part of the molecular structure of myelin. This scenario of "mistaken identity" may explain much of the origin of MS and help to determine how the disease can be prevented from occurring in susceptible people.

An interesting sideline to the concept of molecular mimicry has been a recent focus on the relationship between MS and vaccination of humans to prevent the serious, and potentially fatal, liver disease hepatitis B. Hepatitis B viral infections are not all that common in the general population in the Western world, but occur more often among health-care workers in the West and among the population more generally in the developing world. The disease, and its potentially serious or fatal consequences, can be effectively prevented with a specific vaccination against hepatitis B virus. But there is a degree of molecular mimicry among the virus, the vaccine, and some proteins in myelin, leading to the speculation that a hepatitis B vaccination might result in damage to myelin and lead to the development of MS. Some controversial epidemiologic research has suggested that those who are vaccinated are more likely to develop MS later on than those who are not vaccinated. But there is by no means a clear indication that hepatitis B vaccination and "molecular mimicry" between this (or any) vaccine and myelin is related to development of MS. Indeed, given the serious, life-threatening consequences of a hepatitis B infection in humans, most physicians, governmental health-care systems, and patients accept the necessity of hepatitis B vaccination.

Glial Cell Research—What Is Damaged? What Can Be Repaired?

The symptoms of MS are directly due to inflammation and breakdown of myelin and cells that make myelin—called *oligodendrocytes*—a type of glial cell in the brain and spinal cord of the CNS. Most likely as a secondary (but still early) process, nerve fibers that are wrapped and insulated by myelin also are often damaged in MS. The biology of oligodendrocytes and other glial cells in the CNS is, therefore, a vital and expanding area of research. This includes study of how oligodendrocytes develop and form myelin in early stages of life, how they are affected by immune system responses, how the nervous system responds when myelin is lost, how scars are formed when myelin is lost, and what the potential is for myelin regeneration and recovery.

Basic biochemical studies of myelin using increasingly sophisticated techniques have closely analyzed nervous system tissue in people with MS, and such studies are used to determine if there are any abnormalities in the myelin or oligodendrocytes that might make these tissues and cells vulnerable to immune system attack. Historically, biochemical and anatomic research have repeatedly demonstrated that myelin, or white matter, is "normal" in individuals with MS, suggesting that the autoimmune attack in MS is truly a question of immune cells not recognizing normal self tissue. However, by the mid-1990s, a new technology stemming from magnetic resonance imaging (MRI), called *magnetic resonance spectroscopy* (MRS), began to show that normal-appearing white matter (myelin) in the brains of people with MS may actually have subtle abnormalities. It is not clear if these subtle imaging signals truly reveal myelin tissues or oligodendrocytic cells that are potentially vulnerable to immune attack or whether such signals are a result of a very early, previously undetected disease process. Cause and effect here, as elsewhere in biomedical research, is difficult to sort out. But such studies show not only the power of newer technologies but also the need to constantly reassess scientific beliefs and facts. We still need to consider, therefore, that there may be inherent abnormalities in white matter and myelin in individuals who develop MS and that the immune response directed against such abnormal tissue may be more appropriate than we previously believed—that is, they are not truly self.

For many decades, it was believed that myelin in the CNS could not be regenerated after it was damaged or lost in adults. This belief was shattered by finding in the early 1980s that there was a degree of new myelin development in individuals whose brains showed extensive immune system damage and scarring due to MS. This myelin regeneration was weak, slow, and insufficient to overcome the devastation caused by the disease, but it provided new hope that myelin could be repaired.

Primed by this relatively recent knowledge that damaged CNS oligodendrocytes can regenerate and form new myelin, many laboratories have focused on ways to enhance myelin growth and development in animals and in humans. In most cases of MS, particularly early cases, myelin insulation around nerve fibers is damaged or lost, but the underlying nerve fibers that control functions are intact and probably would be able to function essentially normally if their insulation were restored. This could result in a degree of functional recovery if remyelination could be achieved.

Scientists are pursuing many experimental approaches to meet this challenge. These include identifying the early-stage myelin-making cells in the nervous system, called *oligodendrocyte progenitors*, that are capable, even in adults, of forming new tissue after immune system damage; using "growth factors" to stimulate myelin regeneration; taking advantage of chemical and physical signals that flow between myelin and nerve fibers to stimulate more rapid and efficient myelin growth and nerve regeneration; modulating immune system functions by blocking special immunoglobulins and antibodies that may be inhibiting myelin growth; and transplanting myelin-making cells from healthy donors or from healthy parts of a person's own nervous system to diseased or damaged nervous system sites.

Concepts of transplantation of myelin-making cells or of nerve cells by necessity involve research related to stem cells, including those derived from adult tissues, those derived from fetuses, and those derived from embryos. A key problem in cell or tissue transplantation is the issue of immune system rejection of the transplanted cells and tissues, based on a lack of genetic compatibility of the donor with the recipient—a common occurrence in any tissue (e.g., liver, kidney, heart) transplantation patient. So, the potential of therapeutic cloning of cells, whereby cells or tissues can be created that are genetically identical to the recipient (and thus will not trigger an immune rejection reaction) is also quite relevant.

Research related to stem cells and therapeutic cloning in recent years has been controversial both scientifically and from the perspective of religion, morality, and public policy, and there are no easy answers to the issues that have been raised on any front. However, such research may provide the very best potential, in the long-term, for people living with a variety of debilitating chronic diseases, including MS, where tissues are damaged and might be successfully replaced. The only way to realize that potential is for such research to continue in a careful and carefully monitored fashion.

To date, studies focused on myelin and nerve regeneration and replacement in MS have been largely limited to experimentation in laboratory animals with genetically deficient myelin or animals in which specific myelin lesions have been experimentally produced. Studies using certain immunoglobulins to suppress a theorized immunologic inhibition of myelin growth have been done in humans with MS, with mixed results; more work is planned. One small study that attempted to show remyelination by transplanting peripheral nervous system glial cells into the brains of individuals with MS did not meet with success. But these are the first steps, and over time, more such efforts will be made, and eventually one or more of the cutting-edge techniques may prove to be successful. All of this research provides hope that myelin regrowth and functional recovery for individuals with MS may be possible in the future.

However, no matter what the potential for myelin and nerve fiber regeneration and growth, it is vital to emphasize two key problems related to MS: (1) as long as the immune system problems responsible for myelin destruction in the first place remain unchecked, any efforts at myelin regeneration will be sabotaged by the ongoing immune disease process; and (2) for some individuals, especially those with advanced MS, long-standing nerve fiber damage is likely to be a major component of their disability. Even if myelin can be repaired, for such individuals, repair of nerve fibers will be even more difficult and remote. Thus, research focusing on myelin and nerve regeneration must move hand-in-hand with efforts to stop the underlying immune system process—both to prevent patients from becoming seriously disabled in the first place and to hold in check immune system activity that will simply continue to damage any repaired cells and tissues.

Clinical Research—Treating the Whole Patient

Clinical research directly involves individuals who have MS, not test tubes, not laboratory animals, but individuals living with a chronic disabling disease who experience symptoms, impediments to activities of daily living, and who have to live with consequent impacts on employment, family life, and social interactions. All MS research, no matter how fundamental, is aimed at finding treatments and a cure and at improving the quality of life for people living with MS. Studies in basic immunology, virology, and glial biology, in laboratory test tubes or in animal models of MS, all become applied in the clinic to help us translate such fundamental disease information into studies of people with MS. Clinical trials (see Chapter 10) focus on testing the safety and efficacy of new drugs and agents developed to treat MS and its symptoms (Figure 9–1).

Another important area of clinical research is the refinement and development of new techniques for diagnosis. Such techniques can be used to follow disease progress, particularly the relatively new imaging techniques based on magnetic resonance technology that allow direct observation of lesions in the brain and spinal cord (MRI and related technologies). New developments in analysis of blood, cerebrospinal fluid, and urine also have importance in diagnosis, in tracking disease change over time, and in monitoring the results of experimental clinical studies. All of these technologies played a role in recent refinements of criteria used to diagnosis MS. In particular, the value of imaging and how it should be used has been codified into new MS diagnostic criteria

Figure 9–1. The spectrum of MS research.

Basic Research	→	Clinical Research	→	Patient Management, Care and Rehabilitation Research	→	Health-Care Delivery and Policy Research
aims to		aims to		aims to		aims to
Understand Biologic Mechanisms	→	Apply Basic Understanding to Treat, Prevent, Cure	→	Improve Symptoms and Quality of Life	→	Optimize Delivery of Care and Guide Public Policy

through the widely used McDonald MS Diagnostic Criteria first put forth in 2001 and since refined in 2005 (see Chapter 1).

While new treatments are being developed to help reduce the symptoms and progression of MS, helping individuals and their families cope with the disease, obtain the best possible medical care, and function at the highest possible level in society are essential aspects of research in the areas of psychosocial studies as well as health-care delivery and policy research.

Understanding the psychologic and emotional aspects of MS has become a major focus of research in recent years, as we realize that the brain pathology (as well as day-to-day stress) of the disease creates problems in cognitive (intellectual) and affective (emotional) function. Increased information in these areas is leading to new techniques to help with coping and rehabilitation, as well as specific interventions that can be applied in a clinical setting.

Although not limited to MS, the problems of access to care and services for people with chronic disease are increasingly unwieldy and are becoming the focus of high-quality health-care delivery and policy research. Data gathered from such studies have a direct impact on altering public perception of chronic disease and on changing for the better legislative policy, entitlement programs, and societal policy for all people with disabilities.

Research in MS is broad based and comprehensive, involving all aspects of basic and applied sciences related to biomedicine. Funding for this research traditionally has come from governmental agencies, MS societies in many countries around the world, and, more recently, pharmaceutical and biotechnology companies. To date, the results have been a significantly increased understanding of the disease, new and specific therapies, and significantly enhanced quality of life for people with MS. Basic and applied research are needed more than ever before to close the gaps in our knowledge of MS and move us closer to full treatment, prevention, and cure.

10

||||||||||||||||||||||||||||||||||||||||||||||||||||||||||||||||||||||||||||||||||||||||||||||||||||||||||||||||

Searching for Treatments: The "Ins" and "Outs" of Clinical Trials

A ll biomedical research in multiple sclerosis (MS)—be it the most basic or the most applied—is intended to gather information about the underlying disease process and is ultimately directed toward developing new therapeutic agents that are safe and effective. Beyond research in such fundamental areas as immunology, virology, and neurophysiology, testing new drugs or devices in clinical trials of interventions developed through basic and clinical research is itself a major focus of MS research. The outcome of such research can be treatments that can alter the disease course, prevent the disease from occurring, or improve function in people who already have MS, which together might constitute a functional "cure" for MS. The ultimate research experiment, therefore, is the clinical trial.

A clinical trial is the scientific study of the efficacy and safety of a drug or device for a given disease on people who have that disease. As scientific studies, clinical trials are complex, time consuming, and expensive. They must be done as carefully as any other scientific experiment to ensure that the study results are accurate, reproducible (repeatable by other scientists yielding the same results), and broadly applicable outside the original study population. Poorly done clinical trials that result in misleading conclusions are wasteful at best and potentially dangerous for the intended population needing the treatment.

The Special Problems of MS Trials

Placebo Effects

Clinical trials in MS are particularly difficult to undertake. People with MS generally are highly motivated to search for a treatment or cure for their disease, and this positive motivation can actually interfere with the objective assessment of any drug or device. This often occurs because of a phenomenon known as the *placebo effect*— the tendency to improve simply because of participation in a clinical trial even if no active drug is being administered. A largely psychologic phenomenon, the placebo effect is based in the faith that a given intervention will work even if there is no evidence to support such faith. Working with a sympathetic physician who also strongly believes in the value of an experimental treatment can help to reinforce placebo effects and can give rise to false-positive outcomes in clinical trials.

While considered to be largely psychologic in nature, placebo effects in clinical trials are poorly understood, but clearly have an impact on the biologic responses of a clinical trial study subject. Simply participating in a clinical trial can result in a study subject's increased sense of well-being and increased hope and excitement at the prospect that an experimental agent will have benefit. Such positive psychologic factors can even affect immune system function, thus leading to a real change in immunology that could have a direct impact on this immune-mediated disease. The interaction between psychology, physiology, and disease outcomes in MS is not well understood, but when they occur, they can seem to cause disease improvement—usually temporary unfortunately, since the underlying disease process might be unaffected. Such placebo effects are particularly present when results of experimental treatment rely on self-reporting of symptoms or physical state by a treated patient rather than on the more rigorous objective assessment of performance by an examining physician or on objective laboratory findings.

While important and potentially useful, placebo effects must be carefully separated from a true therapeutic drug effect. Treatments are costly, often inconvenient, and usually have associated side effects. If the impact of a treatment is, in fact, no better than a placebo response, there is no reason to use the drug! So, any useful drug for MS must have an impact that is greater than the placebo effect.

The Natural Disease Variability of Multiple Sclerosis

The high degree of variability in MS makes the design of clinical trials difficult. In any individual, the disease may go through seemingly spontaneous remission and worsening which are unpredictable in occurrence, severity, and duration; no two individuals experience the same problems in the same ways. Spontaneous stabilization in previously progressive disease or a spontaneous remission of symptoms could easily be confused with a drug effect even if the drug is having no impact whatsoever.

Because of this variability, clinical trials for new treatments must include safeguards and design elements that overcome the impact of natural disease variability that is seen over time and within and between individuals. A true drug effect must be separable from the natural variability in disease course.

Understanding the Predicted Drug Effect

New agents for MS are usually chosen for testing because their known or suspected mechanism of action bears some relation to what we know about the disease. For instance, because the disease is widely believed to have an immune system origin, most new agents being tested in MS work through modulating immune functions. However, drugs may have different effects on different MS disease types. Agents that may be predicted to alter the frequency or severity of acute attacks of MS (usually by suppressing or modulating immune-mediated inflammation in the CNS) may have no benefit on longer term progression of disease, which may be due more to tissue degeneration than to inflammation. Thus, clinical trials for acute attacks in MS should include only individuals with well-defined disease relapses; otherwise the results at the end of years of exploration will be uninterpretable. By the same token, results of a study testing the ability of an agent to stop progression of disease would be muddied by the inclusion of patients with relapsing-remitting disease and no progression. Trials must be designed to answer questions on the particular type of disease or symptom for which the experimental agent is predicted—based on its biologic mode of action—to have an effect. The inclusion of individuals with different disease types or without the appropriate symptom problems may result in an incorrect conclusion.

Finally, some drugs may seem to cause improvement but actually only have indirect effects on the MS disease process. This can be the case for agents aimed at treating symptoms of MS (e.g., spasticity, fatigue, depression), in which improvement may be real, but will affect the symptom only and not the underlying disease process. For instance, agents with *psychotropic* effects, such as antidepressants, can help enormously in day-to-day coping with MS for patients who have depression associated with their disease, and such individuals likely will feel and perform better. This could be mistaken for an effect of the medication on the underlying disease process when there really is none at all. This does not make such symptomatic intervention less valuable, but it is important to distinguish between symptom improvement and actual impact on the underlying disease pathology that might come from disease-modifying agents. Understanding the true effect of any drug on the disease process requires a detailed knowledge of the drug's action and careful clinical assessment of effects on the disease.

Availability of Safe and Useful Therapies

Since 1993 a number of treatments for MS have passed the approval process for marketing by the U.S. Food and Drug Administration (FDA) and by other drug regulatory authorities in countries around the world. Relapsing-remitting forms of MS have multiple agents in several different drug classes that have been found to be relatively safe and well tolerated and at least partially effective. Progressive MS with relapses and "worsening MS" can now be treated with drugs that have won regulatory approvals. More agents are being developed for all forms of MS to provide additional therapeutic options for treatable forms of the disease and to find new treatments for types of MS that still remain untreatable (see Chapter 3 for additional information on available therapies.)

The availability of treatments for some forms of MS actually complicates the search for new therapies. Demonstrating that a new agent is safe and effective is most easily done in placebo-controlled studies, in which the experimental agent is given to a group of patients who are compared with an identical group of patients being treated with a placebo preparation—essentially a "sugar pill"—which in fact has no biologic activity. It is preferable that neither patients nor examining physicians know which patient is on active treatment and which is on placebo treatment. In this way, the impact of active treatment can be compared with placebo treatment in a way that keeps subjects and physicians "blinded" to their treatments and thus helps overcome some of the effects of psychologic factors discussed above. Such placebo-controlled trials generally are the most efficient and the least expensive to conduct.

However, the ethics of placebo-controlled clinical trials are questionable if therapy is freely available by prescription. In such a situation, a portion of those enrolled—those who are placed in a placebo group in the trial—would be asked to forego effective treatments for the duration of the new study. This has been specifically addressed in recent revisions of Declaration of Helsinki, an international agreement that sets out guidelines for all human research. The Declaration states that it is an ethical obligation to provide "best available therapy" to all patients involved in research. If an agent is approved for treatment of MS and some patients are asked to withhold from using it so that a placebo-controlled study can be undertaken, that can be seen as a violation of ethics by some investigators, institutional research committees, and patient organizations.

Beyond ethics, there are practical issues involved in conducting placebo-controlled studies: Many patients and physicians simply refuse to participate if there is a risk that some patients will be exposed to a placebo substance—essentially "no therapy"—during the duration of the study, making recruitment and retention of sufficient numbers of patients difficult.

In recent years, a variety of changes in clinical trial study design have been suggested and implemented to help overcome these ethical and practical dilemmas. Some studies only enroll patients who have been clearly informed about the availability of therapy by prescription, and who actively decline to use such therapy; other studies limit the size of placebo groups or limit the duration of time in which a subject is exposed to placebo, offering a "switch" to active therapy at a predetermined time point in the study. Other studies rely increasingly upon patients in "underserved" parts of the world where therapies commonly available in North America or Western Europe are hard to come by. Other clinical trial design innovations that are currently being explored might eliminate placebo groups entirely: by comparing the outcomes of an experimental agent against the readily available treatment; by using a low (but potentially therapeutically valuable) dose of the experimental agent to compare against higher doses; by using placebo group performance in previous MS clinical trials to statistically model "virtual placebo groups" that will significantly reduce or eliminate the need for an actual placebo treatment arm in a study, and so forth. One or more of these might provide a solution to the problem of placebo groups in MS clinical trials in the future; but each will have its own practical and ethical limitations.

Comparison of New Treatments against Available Therapies

New treatments that are being developed need to be at least as good, but hopefully, better (more effective, fewer side effects, easier to use) than those already available. Beyond the practical and ethical issues of placebo-controlled trials noted above, placebo-controlled studies cannot provide comparison information between different agents. The solution is to do direct "head-to-head" clinical trials to determine clinical superiority of one agent over the other. Superiority might be determined by showing increased efficacy of one agent compared to the other, but also by increased safety, increased ease of delivery or compliance, or all of these. For statistical reasons, it is simply not possible to compare the results of placebo-controlled trials of two different agents, each tested alone against placebo, and to say that one is better than the other. All studies have a slightly (or significantly) different patient population, are done in different locations, and are done at different times, all of which make direct comparisons between outcomes of different trials done at different times impossible. However, doing a head-to-head study of the safety and efficacy of a new agent against another already proven effective agent is difficult and expensive. Only a few clinical trials in MS to date have attempted to do so. This means that today we have very little scientific evidence to say how different available therapies for MS compare with each other.

These and other problems associated with MS clinical trials can best be overcome by extremely rigorous experimental designs for the studies. The generally accepted methods of study are time consuming and expensive, and needed innovation is hard to come by, but such rigorous trial designs hold the best chance of obtaining a clear-cut answer about the efficacy and safety of any agent in MS.

Steps in Multiple Sclerosis Clinical Trials

Scientific Rationale: A Primary Requirement

Both scientific rigor and the rules of regulatory agencies such as the FDA, and related agencies in Canada and Europe dictate a set path for development and testing new treatments for human diseases. These include demonstration of biologic relevance, safety, and efficacy in a stepwise fashion that can take many years to accomplish.

The first, and perhaps the most essential step, in the consideration of any new drug or agent for its therapeutic potential in MS is to demonstrate a strong scientific rationale for being tested in this disease. Based on our knowledge of the MS process and on experimental studies of the drug in the laboratory, in animal disease models for MS, or in human disorders with similarities to MS, a scientist will conclude that a drug may have a potential role in the treatment or management of MS. Drugs, or any other substance or device without a scientific rationale related to the known or hypothesized cause of MS, should not even be considered for disease testing. They likely will have no impact on disease outcome and will be wasteful of the time and effort of participating individuals with MS and their physicians, as well as the financial resources required for the study. Many "alternative" therapies can be faulted on this first criterion: a lack of bona fide biologic rationale for even being considered in a disease such as MS.

If a scientific rationale is found, an agent goes through a detailed set of "preclinical" studies, either in laboratory dishes and test tubes (in vitro) or in living animals (in vivo) to better understand the action of the agent, the pharmacologic dynamics of its use, and safety in a setting in which humans are not yet exposed to the agent. Such preclinical testing usually continues even after an agent has been given to humans for evaluation.

"Preliminary" or Phase 1 Studies

Given a strong scientific rationale and acceptable results from preclinical testing in laboratory and animal research, human trials almost always begin with toxicity or safety studies in a very small number of people with the disease. This is a "preliminary" or *phase 1* clinical trial. In such early experiments, physicians usually have little sense of whether the candidate agent is safe for use in humans—the most vital consideration in any medical intervention. In these earliest studies, healthy individuals are often recruited as subjects because they are considered to be least vulnerable and most able to volunteer their time and effort without undue disease-specific pressures. Or, sometimes a few very seriously ill people with the disease in question are asked to participate because these people may find the potential risk of any new untested agent to be worthwhile given the grave nature of their disease. If such studies demonstrate that the agent is safe, a physician may pursue further studies to get a sense of possible efficacy. Phase 1 studies will also often begin to explore different doses or routes of delivery (e.g. oral, injection) of the experimental agent, to help define the safety and tolerability spectrum of the agent.

"Pilot" or Phase 2 Clinical Trials

"Pilot" or *phase 2* studies usually involve larger, statistically relevant numbers of patients (often 20 to 250 or more) with a disease type and severity that seem appropriate to the known or hypothesized drug effect. Key issues in such a study are (1) determining the effectiveness of the drug in halting progression, reducing relapse rate, or improving symptoms and function; (2) obtaining additional information about toxicity and safety; and (3) refining knowledge about the best possible dose and route of delivery.

Such pilot studies aim to be objective in obtaining the required answers. Thus, patient performance on drug may be compared with predrug status (so-called "longitudinal studies") or against the known performance of a similar group of individuals not receiving treatment (a "historical control" study). Even better, they might be compared with an identical group of patients who are on a parallel "control" track but being given sham or placebo treatment (a treatment that looks identical to the actual drug or therapy but is therapeutically inactive) when ethically and practically possible, or with patients who are being actively treated with the best available therapy for that form of disease.

However, because MS can change over time, even with no treatment intervention, longitudinal studies and studies using historical controls usually are unsatisfactory: It is impossible to know whether changes during the trial are due to the test drug or to underlying disease changes that may have occurred anyway. Placebo-controlled (if they can be done ethically and practically) or active treatment controlled studies are preferable even in phase 2 studies.

True objectivity is enhanced in controlled studies if both the patients and the physicians who periodically check for efficacy are "blinded" or "masked" to the treatment status of individual subjects. In other words, neither knows which group of patients is receiving the experimental drug and which group is being given control treatment. Such "double-blinded" studies are hard to achieve, given the fact that many test agents have side effects that may be "unblinding" to the patient or examining physician. But rigorous efforts at blinding are essential to reduce the likelihood of false results due to psychologic responses to the clinical trial itself or to biases about anticipated treatment outcomes among either physicians or patients.

Increasingly, phase 1 and 2 studies are being combined into a "phase 1/2" study to speed the initial assessment of toxicity and efficacy. Magnetic resonance imaging (MRI) to detect the impact of treatment on lesion development in the central nervous system (CNS) is now used as a key outcome in such studies in MS, and often is the primary outcome that is monitored. Most scientists believe the MRI-detected lesions are an excellent marker of disease activity and they reflect the actual disease pathology in the nervous system and since MRI changes tend to occur relatively rapidly compared with more difficult-to-detect clinical changes. Since available therapies for MS all show the ability to reduce accumulation of new lesions detected by MRI, often the first step an investigator takes in evaluating a new treatment is to determine if it, too, can reduce new lesion formation, or at least not result in increased lesions. Of course, MRI outcomes are only applicable in trials in which the expected impact on therapy might be on disease pathology that can be detected by MRI examination. An agent aimed at having an impact on muscle spasticity, for instance, would not be appropriate for a brain MRI-based study! However, for studies where MRI is appropriate as an measure of efficacy, "proof of concept" is the goal, and initial information about dosing, safety, and possible efficacy are the needed outcomes. MRI has largely replaced clinical assessment as the primary mode of analysis in early phase clinical trials.

Results from such phase 1/2 studies can often take several years to obtain. They may or may not show statistical benefit to people receiving drug compared with people receiving control therapy, and may or may not show acceptable levels of side effects and tolerability. An experimental agent usually is abandoned as a possible therapy if there is no benefit, or if there are uncontrollable or dangerous side effects. On the other hand, if the possibility of benefit remains after the study, and side effects are acceptable, a further clinical trial, usually with a primary focus on change in clinical status, will be undertaken to confirm and expand the studies.

"Definitive" or Phase 3 Clinical Trials

"Definitive," "pivotal," or *phase 3* trials usually are the final step toward making a decision about the value of a proposed therapy. As in phase 2 studies, the key questions are efficacy and safety. Large, statistically determined numbers of participants are essential, and the study often is conducted at a number of different sites (so-called "multicenter" trials) and often is international in scope to ensure that the drug can be used in an equivalent fashion by many physicians in many care settings. Rigorous adherence to blinding of patients and examining physicians as well as careful random assignment of patients into treatment and control groups are essential to ensure objectivity. At the conclusion of the study period, when the blinding code is broken and the performance of drug-treated patients can be compared with that of the control group patients, there should be sufficient information to determine if the tested agent is truly safe and effective. Phase 3 studies in MS virtually always track the impact of an experimental agent on measurable clinical change in the patient—for instance, reduction of frequency or severity of relapses or slowing of progression of disability—and additional studies (e.g., imaging or impact of the agent on immune function) might be added as "secondary outcomes" of interest. But to date, the requirement to demonstrate that an agent has an impact on the clinical course, not on a laboratory marker of disease, is paramount for regulatory acceptance.

Recent definitive clinical trials for MS have included as many as 1,500 individuals or more, have involved 50 to 100 or more participating centers, often distributed around the world, and have taken multiple years to complete. These are the "gold standard" studies from which physicians and patients may have the best confidence that the results are sound.

There are variations in these study designs, often depending on the amount of information available about a new drug from the laboratory, from use in other diseases, or from prior use in MS. Not all new agents go through a test phase in animal models of MS (e.g., interferons were not first studied to any extent in animal models of MS because significant amounts of safety data from humans with other diseases were already in hand; such studies have taken place largely after these agents found a place in the treatment armamentarium of MS). And in some cases, phase 2 and phase 3 studies are combined into a single large phase 2/3 study when sufficient information is available from previous studies on dosing and route of delivery. However, the elements and data described are required to determine adequate benefit and safety. These are also the elements and data required by the FDA and similar regulatory bodies in many countries, which closely monitor clinical trials at every step. It is ultimately the regulatory authority's assessment of the efficacy and safety data and the care with which a study is done that determines whether any agent may be marketed as a treatment for MS.

"Postmarketing" or Phase 4 Studies

Once governmental regulatory approval has been granted and a new agent can be marketed and advertised as a treatment for MS, there often is a series of further studies, which are termed "postmarketing" or *phase 4* studies. These usually are designed to collect long-term information about safety and adverse reactions to the agent, to evaluate its continued efficacy over time, to explore the use of the drug for different forms of disease (e.g., an approved drug for progressive MS might be tested in relapsing-remitting disease in a phase 4 analysis or, usually more likely, in an entirely new phase 3 study).

In some cases, regulatory authorities mandate phase 4 studies to collect data that were missing in the definitive analysis and that are important in understanding the use of the new medication. Sometimes the outcome of these mandated phase 4 studies can determine continued marketability of new agents. Should data become available that change the original understanding of the safety and efficacy of the new agent and compromise its use, regulatory authorities may remove the treatment from the market.

Financing Clinical Trials

Drug studies are time consuming and expensive. Such studies most often are supported financially by pharmaceutical and biotechnology companies that invest significant "research and development" resources in these experiments. Grants from the federal government or voluntary health agencies, such as the National Multiple Sclerosis Society and its counterparts around the world, also may fund part or all of the cost of clinical trials. It is rare (and often considered unethical) to request that a patient who volunteers to participate as an experimental subject be asked to pay for that privilege.

Who Participates in Clinical Trials?

The decision for any person with MS to participate in an experimental clinical trial is an intensely personal one and is highly subjective. Since there is always the potential for risk of any untested agent, a potential study participant must be fully informed by the treating physician, who must include a clear assessment of the potential risk factors in the study. Informed consent, including close personal discussion with the physician and nurse as well as required written permission from the study participant, is a legal requirement that protects the rights of all participants.

A true sense of altruism, coupled with a sense of adventure, often characterize those who volunteer to participate in such studies, since participation in either an active treatment or sham group ultimately may help tens of thousands of people with MS. The clinical trial volunteer is a real pioneer and a true hero.

Why Can't Some Patients Participate in Clinical Trials?

An unfortunate dilemma occurs when a person decides that he or she wants to participate in a clinical trial and finds that it is impossible. A frequently asked question is, "Doctor, why can't I be in your clinical trial?"

Clinical trials generally are limited to a relatively small number of individuals, who must be located geographically close to one of the clinical centers where the study is undertaken. Since most studies require intense and frequent clinic visits at specific predetermined times throughout several years, difficulties in travel from home to the clinic may be considered in determining whether someone will be accepted into a study.

The design of trials is such that generally only one type of MS— for instance, relapsing-remitting disease—is involved in the study. This excludes people with any other form of MS. Even within the group of interest, further restrictions, called inclusion and exclusion criteria, will be enforced in virtually all studies: disease limited to a certain duration or a certain level of disability; restricted age of participants; exclusions based on prior medications or participation in previous trials of agents for which there might be dangerous or confusing effects with the new experimental treatment.

For any particular test drug, other restrictions also may apply, depending on the known characteristics of the test medication. There may be prohibitions against pregnancy if an agent might cause harm to a fetus; individuals with other medical conditions not related to MS that may be affected by known characteristics of the test medication may be excluded. These practical factors often can result in an eager patient being refused a place in a new clinical trial.

If this should be the case, disappointed individuals may take some solace from the realization that positive findings from a clinical trial eventually will benefit many, many more people than could ever hope to participate in the initial studies. Everyone will benefit from the time and effort invested by the few.

Where Can I Learn About Ongoing Clinical Trials?

Finding out about clinical trials in MS should be a joint project of the patient and the physician. The network of physicians who organize and participate in MS clinical trials is ever growing, and in consultation with a personal physician, an interested patient usually can learn of any pending studies locally or in nearby communities, often with the assistance of the local branch or chapter of the

National Multiple Sclerosis Society, Multiple Sclerosis Society of Canada, or their over 30 affiliated member organizations around the world. The US National MS Society (www.nationalmssociety.org) has an extensive listing of ongoing and newly recruiting MS clinical trials in the United States and elsewhere, as does the Consortium of MS Centers (www.mscare.org) through its NARCOMS affiliate group; the Multiple Sclerosis International Federation (www.msif.org) carries similar information about trials around the world. Other sources, which might include information about MS clinical trials but are not specific or restricted to MS, include Centerwatch (www.centerwatch.com) and the U.S. Department of Health and Human Services (www.clincaltrials.gov).

In summary, the ultimate goal for research in MS is the development and testing of new therapies for use in the disease. Clinical trials, designed to objectively test efficacy and safety, are difficult and expensive to undertake. While people with MS are always needed to participate in such research, the decision to volunteer is a difficult and personal one, and the practical restrictions involved in conducting clinical trials in MS often exclude many people who would gladly participate. In the end, patients who participate, basic and clinical scientists who find the agents and design the studies, pharmaceutical companies who pursue new treatment directions and fund large-scale trials, and governmental and voluntary health agencies who support basic and clinical research focused on MS worldwide are all partners in ensuring the development of new treatments for individuals affected by MS.

11

||||||||||||||||||||||||||||||||||||||||||||||||||||||||||||||||||||||||||||||||||||||||||||||||||||||||||||||||

How Your Multiple Sclerosis Society Can Help

People with multiple sclerosis (MS) have needs and concerns relative to their diagnosis, many of which are shared by family members and close friends. The issues vary for each individual based on the time since diagnosis, degree of impairment, and family and work situations. Factors such as personality characteristics, previous life events, and learning and coping styles also are involved. The family physician or neurologist is a frequent source of information. While this is certainly appropriate, a medical practice is not an adequate resource to accommodate the extensive nonmedical needs of those with MS, their families, friends, and other concerned persons such as employers, teachers, and health professionals. In North America, the primary resources for addressing nonmedical MS-related needs are the National Multiple Sclerosis Society in the United States and the Multiple Sclerosis Society of Canada. This chapter provides general information about the U.S. and Canadian Societies, as well as the specific ways these organizations can help you.

The National Multiple Sclerosis Society

The National Multiple Sclerosis Society (NMSS) is the only nonprofit organization in the United States that supports national and international research on the prevention, cure, and treatment of MS, with more than $500 million having been expended to date. Equally important, the Society's goals include the provision of nationwide programs to assist people with MS and their families and the provision of information about MS to those with the disease, family members, professionals, and the public. Programs are designed to help people with MS to maintain their independence and lifestyle, with state of the art health-care and other support systems available. The Society's mission—to end the devastating effects of MS—addresses the negative impact of the disease in the present through education and services to support a positive quality of life and into the future through research and advocacy.

The NMSS was founded in 1946 by Sylvia Lawry, whose brother had MS. In her search to learn more about the disease, she found that only two scientists in the country professed any interest in the disease. Ms. Lawry placed an advertisement in the New York Times seeking any information about successful treatments for MS. A number of people who were also touched by MS responded. They had no news of a cure, but asked that Ms. Lawry share whatever helpful information she received. And so the National MS Society was born.

The NMSS has grown to more than 500,000 members, including over 342,000 people who have MS. A 50-state network of chapters provides assistance and education. The home offices in New York City, Denver, and Washington, DC direct MS-related research and advocacy, provide some specific services, and provide support, structure, and guidance for chapters. Policies and national priorities are established by a National Board of Directors, composed of business and professional leaders with a special interest in MS. The Board is assisted by a nationally representative group of individuals with MS, the National Programs Advisory Council. Each local chapter is governed by a Board of Trustees. Staff at both national and chapter levels work in partnership with volunteers and the community to implement the necessary and desired programs. There is an ongoing process of identifying needs and eliciting feedback regarding the value of programs. This involves people with MS, their families, and the professionals who serve them, and provides direction for Society activities.

Philosophy of NMSS Programs

The NMSS and its chapters are committed to empowering people with MS to live as independently as possible within the limits of their disabilities and to the maximum of their capabilities within the least restrictive environment. This goal is achieved through programs, services, and activities that:

- Promote and support knowledge, health, and independence

- Inform and educate people with MS and their families, professionals, public officials, and the general public about MS

- Provide support programs that help people with MS and their families cope with the changes and challenges that MS presents

- Help people gain access to community resources and quality, specialty health care

- Stimulate changes and developments in the community and public policy beneficial to people affected by MS

- Fill gaps in community resources

The Society believes that all people with MS and their families in the United States should have access to certain basic programs and ensures this through its chapter certification process.

All people with MS are offered services without discrimination. Access is not affected by a person's race, color, religion, age, disability, sexual orientation, or the individual's relationship with a chapter. Chapters do hold "targeted" programs to meet the needs of specific groups; for example, education programs for those newly diagnosed, young professionals' groups, and the gay/lesbian community.

The confidentiality of members with MS and their family members ("clients") is strictly maintained. Client status is indistinguishable on the general membership list, and clients receive general Society mailings, including solicitations for support unless a clear request to the contrary is made.

Who Does the NMSS Serve?

The Society's mission reflects our dedication to "end the devastating effects of multiple sclerosis." At the center of chapter programs are people who have MS. Since the disease affects others as well, NMSS clients are all who come to the Society for information and/or professional assistance. The secondary focus of our programs is the MS "family circle"—spouses, children, parents, relatives, and significant others. Coworkers and close friends are included in this circle as well. Family members and significant others can also utilize chapter programs.

The NMSS is the leading source of information on MS for the general public. It also provides education to health professionals, service providers, and community agencies. This information and education can have significant impact on quality of life, increasing access to quality healthcare and community resources, and promoting understanding from others.

Quality of Life Goals

The NMSS organizes services under three main Quality of Life Goals: MS Knowledge, Health, and Independence. Specific services are addressed within this framework.

Knowledge

The NMSS facilitates the acquisition of essential knowledge about MS by providing information and education to clients, families, professionals, and the public.

KNOWLEDGE OF MS BY CLIENTS AND FAMILIES, PROFES-SIONALS, AND THE PUBLIC Information is the first and most frequent request the NMSS receives from people with MS. Client surveys consistently request more information about MS: symptoms, diagnosis, programs, treatment, research, and related issues such as employment, health insurance, disability rights, and family issues.

Seeking information about MS is usually a first step in the coping process. Getting accurate up-to-date information can assist you to make informed decisions, become aware of needs and resources, and take some control over this unpredictable and complex disease. One of the main functions of the NMSS is to serve as the repository of the most current and accurate information on MS. This includes:

- Information can be obtained by calling 1-800-FIGHT-MS (1-800-344-4867).

- Internet Web site with updated information about treatments, current research, and programs (http://www.nationalmssociety.org).

- *Knowledge Is Power* educational program (serial mailings) for people newly diagnosed with MS and their families, available through all chapters or on the Web site.

- *Moving Forward* group educational program for people newly diagnosed with MS and their families.

- Educational programs on various topics throughout the year.

- Annual national education program.

- Booklets, articles, and information sheets on MS-related topics (see Resources).

- Lending library of books, audio- and/or videotapes, with mail access.

- *Inside* MS national bimonthly magazine and chapter newsletter quarterly or more often.

Health

The NMSS helps people with MS to achieve optimal health physically, emotionally, and in their relationships.

PHYSICAL HEALTH   People with MS must deal with concerns about physical impairments related to the disease and their impact on general physical health. NMSS programs and services address physical health needs by:

- Promoting state of the art MS health care and facilitating access for people with MS through formal affiliations with MS clinical facilities and professional education programs

- Providing referrals to neurologists, physical therapists, and other medical/rehabilitation professionals knowledgeable about MS

- Swimming and other exercise programs sponsored or cosponsored by some chapters or referral to existing programs in the community

- Wellness programs

- Affiliation with local MS clinical facilities to facilitate access to, and coordination of, health services

- Participation in local and national advocacy issues related to physical health, for example, health insurance reform, through Action Alert Network. (Call your local chapter to join or sign up on the Society's Web site.)

EMOTIONAL HEALTH   Emotional health is a state of psychological well being, including an individual's adaptive capacities. It is demonstrated by successful interactions with others and with the social environment. Difficulties with adaptation to a chronic illness are normal and respond favorably to a variety of interventions.

Although NMSS chapters are not primarily mental health agencies, we can help individuals and their significant others in their adaptation to chronic illness. Chapters provide short-term counseling: defined as "reflective listening and problem solving." The social isolation that often results from having a chronic illness can be reduced through peer relationships and group programs that bring people together.

Assistance with problem solving, including:

- *"Someone to Listen"* peer support program, which meets the second most requested service—to speak with another person who has MS. "Peers" are specially trained to provide information and support to the person with MS.

- Local counselor/therapist referrals.

- Self-help groups—leaders have often received group leadership training through the Society.

- Peer support programs.

FAMILY SUPPORT   Families of people with MS are important to the NMSS, which has formally adopted the Family Service America, Inc. definition of family: "A family consists of two or more people, whether living together or apart, related by blood, marriage, adoption, or commitment to care for one another."

This definition highlights the inclusion of all varieties of family configurations. The NMSS recognizes the enormous, ongoing stress that the entire family experiences, as well as the critical support provided by the family to the person with MS. Programs emphasize the strengths of the family and bolster these strengths by offering education and other means of support and assistance.

The NMSS sponsors a variety of family programs that combine education, counseling, and social activities. Some chapters have family counseling programs, referrals to experienced community counselors in others. The *Children with MS* program provides support, networking, education, and counseling for children/teens with MS and their parents (call the Denver home office: 303-813-6623).

Independence

The National Multiple Sclerosis Society is committed to promoting the highest possible level of independence for people with MS.

INDEPENDENT LIVING AND ACCESSIBILITY   The NMSS can provide referrals to centers for independent living, equipment vendors, accessible housing, and others.

All chapter offices and program locations are accessible to people with disabilities.

EMPLOYMENT   Referrals and consultations are available to help people continue employment despite MS-related obstacles.

LONG-TERM CARE SERVICES   Programs are available to help people who are moderately to severely limited by MS-related disability receive necessary personal services and other assistance.

The Multiple Sclerosis Society of Canada

Founded in 1948, the Multiple Sclerosis Society of Canada has a membership of 28,000, with seven regional divisions and more than 120 chapters. The head office is located in Toronto, Ontario and division offices are located in Dartmouth, Montreal, Toronto, Winnipeg, Regina, Edmonton, and Vancouver. The mission is "to be a leader in finding a cure for MS and enabling people affected by MS to enhance their quality of life." The Multiple Sclerosis Society of Canada funds a research program totaling about $6 million annually.

Client Services

The Multiple Sclerosis Society of Canada provides a wide variety of programs and services for those affected by multiple sclerosis. These include the following.

INFORMATION AND REFERRAL

- MS Society of Canada publications
- ASK MS and National Information Resource Centre
- Lending libraries
- Information and referrals over the phone or by email

EDUCATION

- Conferences and workshops

SUPPORT

- Individual advocacy
- Support and self-help groups
- Recreation and social programs

ADVOCACY

Helping individuals with MS obtain needed services

FUNDING

- Equipment purchase or loan programs

- Special assistance programs

Services vary across the country depending on the kind of provincial government and community programs available, since the MS Society does not duplicate services available through other sources. The Society currently spends nearly $9 million annually on services and education programs for people who have MS, their family members, and all others affected by MS.

Awareness Activities

The Multiple Sclerosis Society of Canada is firmly committed to informing Canadians about MS and how they can join the fight against MS. The national office coordinates an overall public awareness campaign that is complemented by division and chapter activities.

Government Relations/Social Action

The Multiple Sclerosis Society of Canada works with people who have MS to ensure that they have the opportunity to participate fully in all aspects of life. Volunteers across the country endeavor to change government policies at all levels, private industry practices, and public attitudes in ways that will positively benefit people with MS.

Fund Raising

The Multiple Sclerosis Society of Canada has total revenues of nearly $25 million annually net. The funds are used to support research, client services, public education, social action, and volunteer resources. Most of this income comes from public donations, bequests, and special fund-raising programs conducted by the Canadian MS Society. The major fund raising programs are the MS Carnation Campaign, the RONA MS Bike Tour, the MS Read-A-Thon, the Super Cities WALK for MS, the direct marketing program, and major gifts/ planned giving.

History

A small group of dedicated volunteers in Montreal founded the Multiple Sclerosis Society of Canada in 1948 after contact with the newly established National Multiple Sclerosis Society in the United States. Support of MS research begin in 1949.

Headquarters for the Society remained in Montreal until the mid-1960s, when the offices were moved to Toronto. Other advances came with the establishment of regional divisions; there are now seven divisions across Canada from coast to coast. The Multiple Sclerosis International Federation, of which the Canadian Society is a charter member, was established in 1967.

Multiple Sclerosis Society Division Offices

Alberta Division
Victory Centre
11203-70 Street
Edmonton, AB
T5B 1T1
780-463-1190

Atlantic Division
71 Ilsley Avenue
Unit 12
Dartmouth, NS
B3B 1L5
902-468-8230

British Columbia Division
1501-4330 Kingsway
Burnaby, BC
V5H 4G7
604-689-3144

Manitoba Division
141 Bannatyne Avenue
Suite 400
Winnipeg, MB
R3B 0R3
204-943-9595

Ontario Division
175 Bloor Street East
Suite 700, North Tower
Toronto, ON
M4W 3R9
416-922-6065

Quebec Division
666 Sherbrooke Street
 West, Suite 1500
Montreal, PQ
H3A 1E7
514-849-7591

Saskatchewan Division
150 Albert Street
Regina, SK
S4R 2N2
306-522-5600

National Office
175 Bloor Street East
Suite 700, North Tower
Toronto, ON
M4W 3R8
416-922-6065

Call toll-free in Canada 1-800-268-7582.

MS Clinics

The Multiple Sclerosis Society of Canada is proud to work with a network of specialized MS clinics across the country. Clinic services vary, but most offer a wide range services, delivered by a multidisciplinary health-care team. These services usually include:

• Expert diagnostic and treatment services for people with MS

• Clinical research, especially in the area of MS treatment options

• Educational and support programs for people with MS and their families and caregivers

To learn more about the clinic in your area and the services it provides, contact the clinic directly.

British Columbia
Fraser Health MS Clinic
Burnaby Hospital
Burnaby, BC
604-412-6405

MS Clinic
Kelowna General Hospital
2268 Pandosy Street
Kelowna, BC V1T 1T2
250-862-4225

MS Clinic
Prince George Regional Hospital
2000 15th Avenue
Prince George, BC V2M 1S0
250-565-2304

MS Clinic
UBC Purdy Pavillion G33
2211 Westbrook Mall
Vancouver, BC V6T 2B5
604-822-7131

Vancouver Island MS Clinic
1952 Bay Street, South 1
Victoria, BC V8R 1J8
250-370-8398

Alberta
Multiple Sclerosis Program
Foothills Hospital
Clinic: SSB
2403 29th St. NW
Calgary, AB T2N 2T9
403-944-4253

MS Clinic
9-101 Clinical Sciences
University of Alberta
Edmonton, AL T6G 2G3
780-492-6298

MS Clinic
Red Deer Regional Hospital
Centre
Red Deer, AB
403-343-4674

Saskatchewan
MS Clinic
Saskatoon City Hospital
Room 33- 7th Floor
701 Queen St.
Saskatoon, SK S7K 0M7
306-655-8447

Manitoba
MS Clinic
Health Sciences Centre
GE217-820 Sherbrook St.
Winnipeg, MB R3A 1R9
204-787-5111

Ontario
MS Clinic
Hamilton Health Sciences Corp.
McMaster Site
Box 2000, Station A
Hamilton, ON L8N 3Z5
905-521-2100 ext. 76073

Kingston
MS Clinic
Kingston General Hospital
Connell 7
76 Stuart Street
Kingston, ON K7L 2V7
613-548-2308

London
MS Clinic
London Health Sciences Centre
University Campus
339 Windermere Road
London, ON N6A 5A5
519-663-3697

Ottawa
MS Research Clinic
The Ottawa Hospital – General
Campus
Room 6371, 501 Smyth Road
Ottawa, ON K1H 8L6
613-737-8532

Toronto
Elkie Adler MS Clinic
Sunnybrook and Women's
College Health Science Centre
2075 Bayview Ave.
Toronto, ON M4N 3M5
416-480-5756

MS Clinic
St. Michael's Hospital
30 Bond St., 3-D South

Toronto, ON M5B 1W8
416-864-5377

Pediatric MS Clinic
The Hospital for Sick Children
555 University Avenue
Toronto, ON M5G 1X8
416-813-8133
(Patients must be under 18
years of age)

MS Clinic
St. Joseph's Care Groups
Thunder Bay, ON

Quebec
MS Clinic of L'Estrie
3001 12th Ave. Nort
Fleurimont, QC J1H 5N4
819-346-1110, ext. 14078

MS Clinic
Neuro Rive-Sud
4896 Taschereau Blvd.
Ste. 250
Greenfield Park, QC J4V 2J2
450-672-1931

MS Clinic
Outaouais Vallees de
l'Outaouais Hospital
Pavillon de Hull
116 Lionel-Hemond Blvd.
Hull, QC J8Y 1W7
819-595-6000, ext. 5412

Montreal
MS Clinic
Hospital Notre-Dame
1560 Sherbrooke St. East
3 E Pavillion Deschamps
   H-3135
Montreal, PQ H2L 4M1
514-890-8212

Quebec
MS Clinic
IRDPQ, Clinique
neuromusculaire
525 Hamel Blvd., Suite D-107
Quebec, PQ G1M 2S8
418-529-9141, ext. 6250

Atlantic
Dalhousie MS Research Unit
Centre for Clinical Research
West Annex, Mackenzie Bldg.
5788 University Ave.,
   Room #114
Halifax, NS B3H 1V8
902-422-7817

St. John's
MS Clinic
Division of Neurology
Health Sciences Centre
300 Prince Philip Drive
St. John's, NF A1B 3V6
1-800-563-0495
709-777-6594

Glossary

ACTIVITIES OF DAILY LIVING (ADLs)
Activities of daily living include any daily activity a person performs for self-care (feeding, grooming, bathing, dressing), work, home-making, and leisure. The ability to perform ADLs is often used as a measure of ability/disability in MS.

ACUTE
Having rapid onset, usually with recovery; not chronic or long-lasting.

ANTIBODIES
Proteins of the immune system that are soluble (dissolved) in blood serum or other body fluids and which are produced in response to bacteria, viruses, and other types of foreign antigens. *See* Antigen.

ANTICHOLINERGIC
Refers to the action of certain medications commonly used in the management of neurogenic bladder dysfunction. These medications

inhibit the transmission of parasympathetic nerve impulses and thereby reduce spasms of smooth muscle in the bladder.

ANTIGEN

Any substance that triggers the immune system to produce an antibody; generally refers to infectious or toxic substances. See Antibodies.

ASSISTIVE DEVICES

Any tools that are designed, fabricated, and/or adapted to assist a person in performing a particular task, e.g., cane, walker, shower chair, adapted kitchen utensils, etc.

ATAXIA

The incoordination and unsteadiness that result from the brain's failure to regulate the body's posture and the strength and direction of limb movements. Ataxia is most often caused by disease activity in the cerebellum.

AUTOIMMUNE DISEASE

An immune system malfunction in which the body's immune system causes illness by mistakenly attacking healthy cells, organs, or tissues in the body. Multiple sclerosis is believed to be an autoimmune disease, along with systemic lupus erythematosus, rheumatoid arthritis, scleroderma, and many others.

AUTONOMIC NERVOUS SYSTEM

The part of the nervous system that regulates "involuntary" vital functions, including the activity of the cardiac (heart) muscle, smooth muscles (e.g., of the bladder and bowel), and glands.

AXON

The extension of a nerve cell that conducts impulses to other nerve cells or muscles.

B CELL

A type of lymphocyte (white blood cell) manufactured in the bone marrow that makes antibodies.

BABINSKI REFLEX
A neurologic sign in MS in which stroking the outside sole of the foot with a pointed object causes an upward (extensor) movement of the big toe rather than the normal (flexor) bunching and downward movement of the toes. *See* Sign.

BLOOD-BRAIN BARRIER
A semipermeable cell layer around blood vessels in the brain and spinal cord that prevents large molecules, immune cells, and potentially damaging substances and disease-causing organisms (e.g., viruses) from passing out of the blood stream into the central nervous system (brain and spinal cord). A break in the blood-brain barrier may underlie the disease process in MS.

BRAIN ATROPHY
Shrinkage of the brain that seems to be due, at least in part, to the destruction of myelin and axons. This destruction, and related atrophy, can occur even early in the disease course.

BRAIN STEM
The part of the central nervous system that houses the nerve centers of the head as well as the centers for respiration and heart control. It extends from the base of the brain to the spinal cord.

CATHETER, URINARY
A hollow, flexible tube, made of plastic or rubber, which can be inserted through the urinary opening into the bladder to drain excess urine that cannot be excreted normally.

CENTRAL NERVOUS SYSTEM
The part of the nervous system that includes the brain, optic nerves, and spinal cord.

CEREBELLUM
A part of the brain situated above the brain stem that controls balance and coordination of movement.

CEREBROSPINAL FLUID (CSF)

A watery, colorless, clear fluid that bathes and protects the brain and spinal cord. The composition of this fluid can be altered by a variety of diseases. Certain changes in CSF that are characteristic of MS can be detected with a lumbar puncture (spinal tap), a test sometimes used to help make the MS diagnosis.

CEREBRUM

The large, upper part of the brain, which acts as a master control system and is responsible for initiating thought and motor activity.

CLINICAL FINDING

An observation made during a medical examination indicating change or impairment in a physical or mental function.

CLINICALLY ISOLATED SYNDROME (CIS)

A first neurologic event (e.g., an episode of optic neuritis) that suggests demyelination in the central nervous system, and is accompanied by several "silent" or asymptomatic lesions on MRI that are typical of MS. Individuals with CIS are at high risk for developing clinical definite MS.

CLONUS

A sign of spasticity in which involuntary shaking or jerking of the leg occurs when the toe is placed on the floor with the knee slightly bent. The shaking is caused by repeated, rhythmic, reflex muscle contractions.

COGNITION

High-level functions carried out by the human brain, including comprehension and formation of speech, visual perception and construction, calculation ability, attention (information processing), memory, and executive functions such as planning, problem-solving, and self-monitoring.

COGNITIVE IMPAIRMENT

Changes in cognitive function caused by trauma or disease process. Some degree of cognitive impairment occurs in approximately

50 to 60 percent of people with MS, with memory, information processing, and executive functions being the most commonly affected functions.

COGNITIVE REHABILITATION

Techniques designed to improve the functioning of individuals whose cognition is impaired because of physical trauma or disease. Rehabilitation strategies are designed to improve the impaired function via repetitive drills or practice, or to compensate impaired functions that are not likely to improve. Cognitive rehabilitation is provided by psychologists and neuropsychologists, speech/language pathologists, and occupational therapists. While these three types of specialists use different assessment tools and treatment strategies, they share the common goal of improving the individual's ability to function as independently and safely as possible in the home and work environment.

COMPUTERIZED AXIAL TOMOGRAPHY (CAT SCAN)

A noninvasive diagnostic radiology technique. A computer integrates X-ray scanned "slices" of the organ being examined into a cross-sectional picture.

CONTRACTION

A shortening of muscle fibers and muscle that produce movement around a joint.

COORDINATION

An organized working together of muscles and groups of muscles aimed at bringing about a purposeful movement such as walking or standing.

CORTICOSTEROIDS

See ACTH, Glucocorticoid hormones.

CORTISONE

A glucocorticoid steroid hormone, produced by the adrenal glands or synthetically, that has anti-inflammatory and immune-system suppressing properties. Prednisone and prednisolone also belong to this group of substances used in MS to decrease the duration of attacks.

CRANIAL NERVES
Nerves that carry sensory or motor fibers to the face and neck. Included among this group of twelve nerves are the optic nerve (vision), trigeminal nerve (sensation along the face), vagus nerve (pharynx and vocal cords). Evaluation of cranial nerve function is part of the standard neurologic exam.

DEEP TENDON REFLEXES
The involuntary jerks that are normally produced at certain spots on a limb when the tendons are tapped with a hammer. Reflexes are tested as part of the standard neurologic exam.

DEMYELINATION
A loss of myelin in the white matter of the nervous system.

DIPLOPIA
Double vision, or the simultaneous awareness of two images of the same object that results from a failure of the two eyes to work in a coordinated fashion. Covering one eye will erase one of the images.

DISABILITY
As defined by the World Health Organization, a disability (resulting from an impairment) is a restriction or lack of ability to perform an activity in the manner or within the range considered normal for a human being.

DOUBLE-BLIND CLINICAL STUDY
A study in which none of the participants, including experimental subjects, examining doctors, attending nurses, or any other research staff, know who is taking the test drug and who is taking a control or placebo agent. The purpose of this research design is to avoid inadvertent bias of the test results. In all studies, procedures are designed to "break the blind" if medical circumstances require it.

DYSESTHESIA
Distorted or unpleasant sensations experienced by a person when the skin is touched.

ELECTROENCEPHALOGRAPHY (EEG)
A diagnostic procedure that records, via electrodes attached to various areas of the person's head, electrical activity generated by brain cells.

ELECTROMYOGRAPHY (EMG)
A diagnostic procedure that records muscle electrical potentials through electrodes.

ETIOLOGY
The study of all factors that may be involved in the development of a disease, including the patient's susceptibility, the nature of the disease-causing agent, and the way in which the person's body is invaded by the agent.

EVOKED POTENTIALS (EPs)
Recordings of the nervous system's electrical response to the stimulation of specific sensory pathways (e.g., visual, auditory, general sensory). Evoked potentials can demonstrate lesions along specific nerve pathways whether or not the lesions are producing symptoms, thus making this test useful in confirming the diagnosis of MS.

EXACERBATION
The appearance of new symptoms or the aggravation of old ones (synonymous with attack, relapse, flare-up, or worsening); usually associated with inflammation and demyelination in the brain or spinal cord.

EXPERIMENTAL ALLERGIC ENCEPHALOMYELITIS (EAE)
An autoimmune disease resembling MS that is induced in genetically susceptible research animals. Before testing on humans, a potential treatment for MS may first be tested on laboratory animals with EAE in order to suggest the treatment's efficacy and safety in humans.

EXTENSOR SPASM

A symptom of spasticity in which the legs straighten suddenly into a stiff, extended position. These spasms, which typically last for several minutes, occur most commonly in bed at night or on rising from bed.

FLACCID

A decrease in muscle tone resulting in loose, "floppy" limbs.

FLEXOR SPASM

Involuntary, sometimes painful contractions of the flexor muscles, which pull the legs upward into a clenched position. They often occur during sleep, but can also occur when the person is in a seated position.

FOOD AND DRUG ADMINISTRATION (FDA)

The U.S. federal agency that is responsible for establishing and enforcing governmental regulations pertaining to the manufacture and sale of food, drugs, and cosmetics. Its role is to certify benefits of medication and prevent the sale of impure or dangerous substances. Any new drug that is proposed for the treatment of MS must be approved by the FDA.

FOOT DROP

A condition of weakness in the muscles of the foot and ankle, caused by poor nerve conduction, which interferes with a person's ability to flex the ankle and walk with a normal heel-toe pattern. The toes touch the ground before the heel, causing the person to trip or lose balance.

FRONTAL LOBES

The anterior (front) part of each of the cerebral hemispheres that make up the cerebrum. The back part of the frontal lobe is the motor cortex, which controls voluntary movement; the area of the frontal lobe that is further forward is concerned with learning, behavior, judgment, and personality.

GLUCOCORTICOID HORMONES

Steroid hormones that are produced by the adrenal glands in response to stimulation by adrenocorticotropic hormone (ACTH) from the pituitary. These hormones, which can also be manufactured synthetically (prednisone, prednisolone, methylprednisolone, betamethasone, dexamethasone), serve both an immunosuppressive and an anti-inflammatory role in the treatment of MS exacerbations: they help control overactive immune response and interfere with the release of certain inflammation-producing enzymes.

HANDICAP

As defined by the World Health Organization, a handicap is a disadvantage, resulting from an impairment and disability, that interferes with a person's efforts to fulfill a role that is normal for that person. Handicap is therefore a social concept, representing the social and environmental consequences of a person's impairments and disabilities.

HELPER T-LYMPHOCYTES

White blood cells that are a major contributor to the immune system's inflammatory response against myelin.

IMMUNE SYSTEM

A complex system of cells and dissolvable proteins that protect the body against disease-producing organisms and other foreign invaders.

IMMUNOCOMPETENT CELLS

White blood cells (B- and T-lymphocytes and others) that defend against invading agents in the body.

IMMUNOSUPPRESSION

In MS, a form of treatment that slows or inhibits the body's natural immune responses, including those directed against the body's own tissues. Examples of immunosuppressive treatments in MS include cyclophosphamide, cyclosporine, methotrexate, and azathioprine.

IMPAIRMENT
As defined by the World Health Organization, an impairment is any loss of function directly resulting from injury or disease.

INCIDENCE
The number of new cases of a disease in a specified population over a defined period of time.

INCONTINENCE
The inability to control passage of urine or feces.

INFLAMMATION
A tissue's immunologic response to injury, characterized by mobilization of white blood cells and antibodies, swelling, and fluid accumulation.

INTENTION TREMOR
Rhythmic shaking that occurs in the course of a purposeful movement, such as reaching to pick something up or bringing an outstretched finger in to touch one's nose.

INTERFERON
A group of immune system proteins, produced and released by cells infected by a virus, which inhibit viral multiplication by modifying the body's immune response. Several interferons have been approved by the Food and Drug Administration for treatment of relapsing-remitting MS.

LUMBAR PUNCTURE
A diagnostic procedure that uses a hollow needle to penetrate the spinal canal to remove cerebrospinal fluid for analysis. This procedure is used to examine the cerebrospinal fluid for changes in composition that are characteristic of MS (e.g., elevated white cell count, elevated protein content).

LYMPHOCYTE
A type of white blood cell that is part of the immune system. Lymphocytes can be subdivided into two main groups: B-lymphocytes, which

originate in the bone marrow and produce antibodies; T-lymphocytes, which are produced in the bone marrow and mature in the thymus. Helper T-lymphocytes heighten immune responses; suppressor T-lymphocytes suppress them and seem to be in short supply during an MS exacerbation.

MACROPHAGE
A white blood cell with scavenger characteristics that ingests and destroys foreign substances, such as bacteria and cell debris.

MAGNETIC RESONANCE IMAGING (MRI)
A diagnostic procedure that produces visual images of body parts without the use of X-rays. An important diagnostic tool in MS, MRI makes it possible to visualize and count lesions in the white matter of the brain and spinal cord.

MINIMAL RECORD OF DISABILITY (MRD)
A standardized method for quantifying the clinical status of a person with MS. The MRD is made up of five parts: demographic information; the Neurological Functional Systems, which assign scores to clinical findings for each of the various neurologic systems in the brain and spinal cord (pyramidal, cerebellar, brain stem, sensory, visual, mental, bowel and bladder); the Disability Status Scale, which gives a single composite score for the person's disease; the Incapacity Status Scale, which is an inventory of functional disabilities relating to activities of daily living; the Environmental Status Scale, which provides an assessment of social handicap resulting from chronic illness. The MRD assist doctors and other professionals in assessing the impact of MS and in planning and coordinating the care of people with MS.

MONOCLONAL ANTIBODIES
Laboratory-produced antibodies, which can be designed to react against a specific antigen in order to alter the immune response.

MOTOR NEURONS
Nerve cells of the brain and spinal cord that enable movement of muscles in various parts of the body.

MUSCLE TONE

A characteristic of a muscle brought about by the constant flow of nerve stimuli to that muscle. Abnormal muscle tone can be defined as: hypertonus (increased muscle tone, as in spasticity); hypotonus (reduced muscle tone (flaccid paralysis); atony (loss of muscle tone). Muscle tone is evaluated as part of the standard neurologic exam in MS.

MYELIN

A fatty white coating of nerve fibers in the central nervous system, composed of lipids (fats) and protein. Myelin serves as insulation and as an aid to efficient nerve fiber conduction. When myelin is damaged in MS, nerve fiber conduction is faulty or absent.

MYELIN BASIC PROTEIN

A protein comprising about 30 percent of all myelin of the central nervous system that may be found in higher than normal concentrations in the cerebrospinal fluid of individuals with MS and other diseases that damage myelin. Some believe myelin basic protein is an antigen against which autoimmune responses are triggered in MS.

MYELITIS

An inflammatory disease of the spinal cord. In transverse myelitis, the inflammation spreads across the tissue of the spinal cord, resulting in a loss of its normal function to transmit nerve impulses up and down, as though the spinal cord had been severed.

NERVE

A bundle of nerve fibers (axons). Fibers are either afferent (leading toward the brain and serving in the perception of sensory stimuli of the skin, joints, muscles, and inner organs) or efferent (leading away from the brain and mediating contractions of muscles or organs).

NERVOUS SYSTEM

Includes all of the neural structures in the body: the central nervous system consists of the brain, spinal cord, and optic nerves; the peripheral nervous system consists of the nerve roots and nerves throughout the body.

NEUROGENIC BLADDER
Bladder dysfunction associated with neurologic malfunction in the nervous system and characterized by a failure to empty, failure to store, or a combination of the two. Symptoms that result from these three types of dysfunction include urinary urgency, frequency, hesitancy, nocturia, and incontinence.

NEUROLOGIST
Physician who specializes in the diagnosis and treatment of conditions related to the nervous system.

NEURON
The basic nerve cell of the nervous system. A neuron consists of a nucleus within a cell body and one or more processes (extensions) called dendrites and axons.

OCCUPATIONAL THERAPIST (OT)
Occupational therapists assess functioning in activities of everyday living that are essential for independent living, including dressing, bathing, grooming, meal preparation, writing, and driving.

OLIGOCLONAL BANDS
A diagnostic sign indicating abnormal levels of certain antibodies in the cerebrospinal fluid; seen in approximately 90 percent of people with multiple sclerosis, but not specific to MS.

OLIGODENDROCYTE
A cell in the central nervous system that is responsible for making and supporting myelin.

OPTIC NEURITIS
Inflammation or demyelination of the optic (visual) nerve with transient or permanent impairment of vision and occasionally pain.

ORTHOSIS

A mechanical appliance (such as a leg brace or splint) that is specially designed to control, correct, or compensate for impaired limb function.

PARESTHESIA

A sensation of burning, prickling, tingling, or creeping on the skin that is often seen in MS.

PAROXYSMAL SYMPTOMS

Symptoms that have sudden onset, apparently in response to some kind of movement or sensory stimulation, last for a few moments, and then subside. Paroxysmal symptoms tend to occur frequently in those individuals who have them, and follow a similar pattern from one episode to the next. Examples of paroxysmal symptoms include acute episodes of trigeminal neuralgia (sharp facial pain), tonic seizures (intense spasm of limb or limbs on one side of the body), dysarthria (slurred speech often accompanied by loss of balance and coordination), and various paresthesias (sensory disturbances ranging from tingling to severe pain).

PHYSIATRIST

Physicians who specialize in the rehabilitation of physical impairments.

PHYSICAL THERAPIST (PT)

Physical therapists evaluate and improve movement and function of the body, with particular attention to physical mobility, balance, posture, fatigue, and pain.

PLACEBO

An inactive compound designed to look just like a test drug in a clinical drug study as a means of assessing the benefits and liabilities of the test drug taken by experimental group subjects.

PLACEBO EFFECT

An apparently beneficial result of therapy that occurs because of the patient's expectation that the therapy will help, in the absence of any real treatment.

PLAQUE
An area of inflamed or demyelinated central nervous system tissue.

POSTURAL TREMOR
Rhythmic shaking that occurs when the muscles are tensed to hold an object or stay in a given position.

PREVALENCE
The number of all new and old cases of a disease in a defined population at a particular point in time.

PRIMARY PROGRESSIVE MS
A clinical course of MS characterized from the beginning by progressive disease, with no plateaus or remissions, or an occasional plateau and very short-lived, minor improvements.

PROGNOSIS
Prediction of the future course of the disease.

PROGRESSIVE-RELAPSING MS
A clinical course of MS that shows disease progression from the beginning, but with clear, acute relapses along the way.

PSEUDO-EXACERBATION
A temporary aggravation of disease symptoms, sometimes resulting from an elevation in body temperature or other stressor (e.g., an infection, severe fatigue, constipation), that disappears once the stressor is removed. A pseudo-exacerbation involves temporary flare-ups of prior or existing symptoms rather than new disease activity or progression.

PYRAMIDAL TRACTS
Motor nerve pathways in the brain and spinal cord that connect nerve cells in the brain to the motor cells located in the cranial, thoracic, and lumbar parts of the spinal cord. Damage to these tracts causes spastic paralysis or weakness.

REFLEX

An involuntary response of the nervous system to a stimulus, such as the stretch reflex, which is elicited by tapping a tendon with a reflex hammer, resulting in a contraction. Increased, diminished, or absent reflexes can be indicative of neurologic damage, including MS, and are therefore tested as part of the standard neurologic exam.

RELAPSE

Also known as attack, flare-up, or exacerbation. The appearance of new symptoms or the aggravation of old ones, lasting at least 24 hours; usually associated with inflammation and demyelination in the brain or spinal cord.

RELAPSING-REMITTING MS

A clinical course of MS that is characterized by clearly defined, acute attacks (relapses) with full or partial recovery and no disease progression between attacks.

REMISSION

A lessening in the severity of symptoms or their temporary disappearance during the course of the illness.

REMYELINATION

The repair of damaged myelin. Myelin repair occurs spontaneously in MS but very slowly.

SCLEROSIS

Hardening of tissue. In MS, sclerosis is the replacement of lost myelin around CNS nerve cells with scar tissue.

SECONDARY PROGRESSIVE MS

A clinical course of MS that initially is relapsing-remitting and then becomes continuously progressive at a variable rate, with or without occasional relapses along the way. The disease-modifying medications are thought to provide benefit for those who continue to have relapses.

SENSORY
Related to bodily sensations such as pain, smell, taste, temperature, vision, hearing, and position in space.

SIGN
An objective physical problem or abnormality identified by the physician during the neurologic examination, including altered eye movements and other changes in the appearance or function of the visual system; altered reflexes; weakness; spasticity; sensory changes.

SPASTICITY
Abnormal increase in muscle tone, manifested as a springlike resistance of an extremity to moving or being moved.

SPHINCTER
A circular band of muscle fibers that tightens or closes a natural opening of the body, such as the external anal sphincter, which closes the anus, and the internal and external urinary sphincters, which close the urinary canal.

STEROIDS
See Glucocorticoid hormones.

SYMPTOM
A subjectively perceived problem or complaint reported by the patient. In multiple sclerosis, common symptoms include visual problems, fatigue, sensory changes, weakness or paralysis of limbs, tremor, lack of coordination, poor balance, bladder or bowel changes, and psychological changes. *See* Sign.

TONIC SEIZURE
An intense spasm that lasts for a few minutes and affects one or both limbs on one side of the body. Like other types of paroxysmal symptoms in MS, these spasms occur abruptly and fairly frequently in those individuals who have them, and are similar from one brief episode to the next. The attacks may be triggered by movement or occur spontaneously. *See* Paroxysmal symptom.

TRIGEMINAL NEURALGIA
Lightning-like, acute pain in the face caused by demyelination of nerve fibers at the site where the sensory (trigeminal) nerve root for that part of the face enters the brain stem.

URINARY FREQUENCY
Need or urge to urinate more frequently than normal due to small hyperactive bladder.

URINARY HESITANCY
The inability to void urine spontaneously even though the urge to do so is present.

URINARY URGENCY
The inability to postpone urination once the need to void has been felt.

VERTIGO
A dizzying sensation of the environment spinning, often accompanied by nausea and vomiting.

Additional Readings

Books from Demos Medical Publishing

Bowling A. *Alternative Medicine and Multiple Sclerosis,* 2001.

Coyle PK, Halper J. *Meeting the Challenges of Progressive Multiple Sclerosis,* 2001.

Davis A. *My Story: A Photographic Essay on Life with Multiple Sclerosis,* 2004.

Giffels JJ. *Clinical Trails: What You Should Know Before Volunteering to Be a Research Subject,* 1996.

Kalb R, (ed.) *Multiple Sclerosis: The Questions You Have; The Answers You Need* (3rd ed.), 2004.

Kalb R. *Multiple Sclerosis: A Guide for Families* (3rd ed.), 2006.

Kraft GH. Catanzaro M. *Living with Multiple Sclerosis: A Wellness Approach* (2nd ed.), 2000.

Kramer D. *Life on Cripple Creek; Essays on Living with Multiple Sclerosis,* 2003.

Murray J. *Multiple Sclerosis: The History of a Disease,* 2004.

Nichols J. *Women Living with Multiple Sclerosis,* 1999.

Nichols J. *Living Beyond Multiple Sclerosis: A Women's Guide*, 2000.

Northrop D. *Cooper S, Calder K. Health Insurance Resources: A Guide for People with Chronic Disease and Disability* (2nd ed.), 2007.

Perkins L, Perkins S. *Multiple Sclerosis: Your Legal Rights* (2nd ed.), 1999.

Rogers, J. *The Disabled Woman's Guide to Pregnancy and Birth*, 2006.

Rumrill PD, Jr. (ed.). *Employment Issues and Multiple Sclerosis*, 1996.

Schapiro RT. *Symptom Management in Multiple Sclerosis* (5th ed.), 2007.

Other Books

Baldacci S. *A Sundog Moment*. Warner Faith, 2004.

Barrett M. *Sexuality and Multiple Sclerosis*. 3rd ed. Toronto: Multiple Sclerosis Society of Canada, 1991.

Barrett S. Jarvis WT, (eds.) *The Health Robbers: A Close Look at Quackery in America*. Buffalo: Prometheus Books, 1993.

Blackstone M. *First Year—Multiple Sclerosis: An Essential Guide for the Newly Diagnosed*. New York: Marlowe and Co., 2002.

Cassileth BR. *The Alternative Medicine Handbook*. New York: W.W. Norton & Co., 1998.

Chapman B. *Coping with Vision Loss: Maximizing What You Can See and Do*. Alameda: Hunter House, 2001.

Cristall B. *Coping When a Parent has Multiple Sclerosis*. New York: Rosen Publishing, 1992. [written for teens].

Donoghue PJ, Siegel ME. *Sick and Tired of Feeling Sick and Tired: Living with Invisible Chronic Illness*. New York: WW Norton, 1992.

Fennell P. *The Chronic Illness Workbook*. New Harbinger Publications, Inc., 2001.

Hill B. *Multiple Sclerosis Q & A: Reassuring Answers to Frequently Asked Questions*. Avery Penguin Putnam, 2003.

James JL. *One Particular Harbor: The Outrageous True Adventures of One Woman with Multiple Sclerosis Living in the Alaskan Wilderness*. Chicago: Noble Press, 1993.

Kalb R, Geisser B, Holland N. *Multiple Sclerosis for Dummies.* New Jersey: John Wiley & Sons, Inc., 2007.

Lander D. *Fall Down Laughing.* Putnam Publishing Group, 2000.

MacFarlane EB. Burstein P. *Legwork: An Inspiring Journey through a Chronic Illness.* New York: Charles Scribner's Sons, 1994.

Pitzele SK. *We Are Not Alone: Learning to Live with Chronic Illness.* New York: Workman Publishing, 1986.

Pitzele SK. *One More Day: Daily Meditations for the Chronically Ill.* Minnesota: Hazelden,1988.

Resources for Rehabilitation. *Making Wise Medical Decisions: How to Get the Information You Need* (2nd ed.) Winchester: Resources for Rehabilitation, 2001.

Russell M. (ed.) *When the Road Turns: Inspirational Stories By and About People with MS.* Health Communications, Inc., 2001.

Spero D. *The Art of Getting Well: A Five-Step Plan for Maximizing Health When You Have a Chronic Illness.* Alameda: Hunter House, 2002.

Strong M. *Mainstay: For the Well Spouse of the Chronically Ill.* Bradford Books, 1997.

Tyler VE. *The Honest Herbal (4th ed.)* New York: Haworth Press, 1998.

Winks C. Semans A. *The Good Vibrations Guide to Sex* (3rd ed.) San Francisco: Cleis Press, 2004.

Wright LM, Leahey M. *Families and Chronic Illness.* Philadelphia: Spring House, 1987.

Yaffe M, Fenwick E, Rosen RC, Kellett JM. *Sexual Happiness for Women: A Practical Approach.* New York: Henry Holt & Co., 1992.

Yaffe M, Fenwick E, Rosen RC, Kellett JM. *Sexual Happiness for Men: A Practical Approach.* New York: Henry Holt & Co., 1992.

Resources

There is a vast array of resources available to help you in your efforts to meet the challenges of multiple sclerosis. This list is by no means a complete one; it is designed as a starting point in your efforts to identify the resources you need. Each resource that you investigate will lead you to others and they, in turn, will lead you to even more.

Information Sources

National Health Information Center (P.O. Box 1133, Washington, D.C. 20013; tel: 800-336-4797; Internet: *www.health.gov/nhic*). The Center maintains a library and a database of health-related organizations. It also provides referrals related to health issues for consumers and professionals.

Electronic Information Sources

There are many sources of information available free through the Internet on the World Wide Web. If you are an experienced "net surfer," switch to your favorite search facility and enter the keywords "MS" or "multiple sclerosis." This will generally give you a listing of dozens of web sites that pertain to MS. Keep in mind, however, that the World Wide Web is a free and open medium; while many of the web sites have excellent and useful information, others may contain highly unusual and inaccurate information. Following is a list of some recommended MS sites available through the Internet. Each of these will provide links to other sites.

Avonex®
http://www.avonex.com/

Betaseron®
http://www.betaseron.com/

CenterWatch Clinical Trials Listing Service™
http://www.centerwatch.com/

CLAMS—Computer Literate Advocates for Multiple Sclerosis
http://www.clams.org/

Consortium of Multiple Sclerosis Centers
http://www.mscare.org/

Copaxone®
http://www.copaxone.com/

The Heuga Program
A program emphasizing health, physical fitness, and psychological well-being
http://www.heuga.org

Infosci
Selected Links on MS
http://www.infosci.org/

International Federation of Multiple Sclerosis Societies/The World of Multiple Sclerosis
http://www.msif.org/

Medicare Information
http://www.medicare.gov

Microsoft Accessibility Technology for Everyone
http://www.microsoft.com/enable/

MS Crossroads
Personal Website of Aapo Halko, Ph.D., mathematician with MS in Finland
http://www.mscrossroads.org

The Multiple Sclerosis Information Gateway
Schering AG, Berlin, Germany
http://www.ms-gateway.com/

Multiple Sclerosis Society of Canada
http://www.mssociety.ca/

Myelin Project
http://www.myelin.org/

National Institute of Neurological Disorders and Stroke
http://www.ninds.nih.gov/

National Library of Medicine
http://www.nlm.nih.gov/

National Multiple Sclerosis Society
http://www.nationalmssociety.org/

National Organization for Rare Disorders
http://www.rarediseases.org/

NARIC—The National Rehabilitation Information Center
http://www.naric.com/

Novantrone®
http://www.novantrone.com

Rebif®
http://www.rebif.com

Resource Materials

The Complete Directory for People with Chronic Illness, 1998–1999, (published by Grey House Publishing, Inc., 185 Millerton Road, P.O. Box 860, Millerton, NY 12546; tel: 800-562-2139; fax: 860-435-3004; e-mail: www.greyhouse.com).

Complete Drug Reference. (Compiled by United States Pharmacopoeia, published by Consumer Report Books, A division of Consumers Union, Yonkers, NY.). This comprehensive, readable, and easy-to-use drug reference includes almost every prescription and non-prescription medication available in the United States and Canada. A new edition is published yearly.

Complete Guide to Prescription and Non-Prescription Drugs. (Written by H. Winter Griffith, M.D., published by The Body Press/Perigee, 200 Madison Avenue, New York, NY 10016, 1995).

Agencies and Organizations

Consortium of Multiple Sclerosis Centers (CMSC) (c/o Holy Name Hospital MS Center, 718 Teaneck Road, Teaneck, NJ 07666; tel: 201-837-0727; Internet: *www.mscare.org*). The CMSC is made up of numerous MS centers throughout the United States and Canada. The Consortium's mission is to disseminate information to clinicians, increase resources and opportunities for research, and advance the standard of care for multiple sclerosis. The CMSC is a multidisciplinary organization, bringing together healthcare professionals from many fields involved in MS patient care.

Department of Veterans Affairs (VA) (810 Vermont Avenue, N.W., Washington, D.C. 20420; tel: 202-273-5400; Internet: *www. va.gov*). The VA provides a wide range of benefits and services to those who have served in the armed forces, their dependents, beneficiaries of deceased veterans, and dependent children of veterans with severe disabilities.

Equal Employment Opportunity Commission (EEOC) (Office of Communication and Legislative Affairs, 1801 L Street, N.W., 10th Floor, Washington, D.C. 20507; tel: 800-669-3362 (to order publications); 800-669-4000 (to speak to an investigator; 202-663-4900; Internet: *www.eeoc.gov*). The EEOC is responsible for monitoring the section of the ADA on employment regulations. Copies of the regulations are available.

Heuga Center (27 Main St., Suite 303, Edwards, CO 81632; tel; 1-800-367-3101; World Wide Web at http://www.heuga.org). The Heuga Center is a non-profit organization dedicated to improving the lives of people and families living with MS through interactive, educational programs unique to any in the world. With an interdisciplinary team of MS experts in fields such as neurology, psychology, occupational, physical and speech therapy, and nutrition, the CAN DO, JUMPSTART, AND OTHER Heuga Center programs offer a supportive, nurturing environment in which participants learn to take control of their lives and their health by focusing on what they "can do" instead of what they cannot. The Center's programs, offered throughout North America, help participants set realistic personal goals construct an individualized lifestyle plan, and gain the strategies and skills necessary to be successful in improving their life. Heuga Center programs also address the needs and education of support partners and family members.

Multiple Sclerosis Society of Canada (250 Bloor Street East, Suite 100, Toronto, ON, M4W 3P9 Canada; tel 416-922-6065; in Canada: 800-268-7582; Internet: www.mssociety.ca). A national organization that funds research, promotes public education, and produces publications in both English and French. They provide an "ASK MS Information System" database of articles on a wide variety of topics including treatment, research, and social services. Regional divisions and chapters are located throughout Canada.

National Multiple Sclerosis Society (NMSS) (733 Third Avenue, New York, NY 10017; tel: 800-FIGHT-MS; Internet: *www.nation-almsssociety.org*). The NMSS is a nonprofit organization that supports national and international research into the prevention, cure, and treatment of MS. The Society's goals include provision of nation-wide services to assist people with MS and their families, and provision of information to those with MS, their families, professionals, and the public. The programs and services of the Society promote knowledge, health, and independence while providing education and emotional support:

- Toll-free access to your by calling 800-FIGHT-MS (800-344-4867).

- Internet Web site with updated information about treatments, current research, and programs (*http://www.nation-almssociety.org*); local home page in many areas.

- Knowledge Is Power—an eight-segment, learn-at-home program (serial mailings) for people newly diagnosed with MS and their families.

- MS Learn Online—online, interactive Web casts on a wide variety of topics.

- Printed materials on a variety of topics available by calling 800-FIGHT-MS (800-344-4867) or in the Library section of the National MS Society Web site at *http://www.nationalms-society.org/library.asp*.

- Educational programs on various topics throughout the year, provided through individual chapters.

- Annual national education conference, provided through individual chapters.

- Swimming and other exercise programs sponsored or co-sponsored by some chapters, or referral to existing programs in the community.

- Wellness programs in some chapters.

United Spinal Association (USA) (75-20 Astoria Boulevard, Jackson Heights, NY 11370; tel: 718-803-3782; Internet: *www.unitedspinal. org*). USA is a private, nonprofit organization dedicated to serving the needs of its members as well as other people with spinal cord injury or disorder. While offering a wide range of benefits to members with spinal cord dysfunction (including hospital liaison, sports and recreation, wheelchair repair, adaptive architectural consultations, research and educational services, communications, and information services), they will also provide brochures and information on a variety of subjects, free of charge to the general public.

Well Spouse Foundation (610 Lexington Avenue, New York, NY 10022-6005; tel: 212-644-1241; 800-838-0879; Internet: *www. wellspouse.org*). An emotional support network for people married to or living with a chronically ill partner. Advocacy for home health and long-term care and a newsletter are among the services offered.

Assistive Technology

Life Enhancement Technologies, LLC (807 Aldo Ave., Suite 101, Santa Clara, CA 95054; tel:408-336-6940; Internet: *www.2bcool. com*). The company manufactures a variety of cooling suits that can be used in management of heat-related symptoms in MS.

Medic Alert Foundation International (2323 Colorado Ave., Turlock, CA 95382; tel: 888-633-4298; 209-668-3333; Internet:

www.medicalert.org). A medical identification tag worn to identify a person's medical condition, medications, allergies and any other important information that might be needed in case of an emergency. A file of the person's health data is maintained in a central database to be accessed by a physician or other emergency personnel who need to know the person's pertinent medical information.

About the Authors

NANCY J. HOLLAND, RN, EdD, MSCN

Dr. Holland is vice president of Clinical Programs at the National Multiple Sclerosis Society in New York City, where she works with national and international leaders in the areas of MS care and rehabilitation. Dr. Holland has been active in the field of MS for over 30 years. She has many years of clinical experience and helped found the first comprehensive MS care center in the US. She is a founding director of the International Organization of MS Nurses and author/editor of more than 60 MS-related articles, chapters, and books, including *Multiple Sclerosis in Clinical Practice, Comprehensive Nursing Care in Multiple Sclerosis, and Multiple Sclerosis: A Self-Care Guide for Wellness.* Dr. Holland serves on many MS advisory boards and is executive editor of *MS in Focus,* a publication of the MS International Federation. She earned a doctorate in higher and adult education from Columbia University, and holds undergraduate and graduate degrees in nursing.

T. Jock Murray, MD

Dr. T. Jock Murray is professor emeritus of Medicine and Neurology at Dalhousie University in Halifax, NS, Canada. He is the former dean of medicine and is chairman emeritus of the American College of Physicians. Although he has had career involvement in medical education, medical history and medical administration, with international awards for lifetime contributions to these areas, his clinical and research area has been multiple sclerosis. He has published over 250 medical papers, held 91 funded research grants and authored seven books. He was a founder of the Consortium of MS Centers and the Canadian Network of MS Centers, and was awarded the Dr. Labe Scheinberg Award for contributions to MS research. He combined his interest in multiple sclerosis and medical history in the recent publication of *Multiple Sclerosis: The History of a Disease*, which was awarded the ForeFront Silver Medal as the best book on history in 2005. He has been awarded three honorary degrees and was made an officer of the Order of Canada.

Stephen Charles Reingold, PhD

Stephen C. Reingold, PhD, is president of Scientific and Clinical Review Associates, LLC., a consulting group that provides strategic guidance in scientific research, pharmaceutical and biotech product development, and clinical trial design and implementation in neurology. He also serves as research counselor for the National Multiple Sclerosis Society (USA).

Dr. Reingold has over 35 years of experience in biomedical research and administration focused on neuroscience. He obtained a Bachelors of Science degree with honors from the University of California, Berkeley, a doctorate in neurophysiology from Cornell University, and undertook postdoctoral research and teaching at Princeton University. Beginning in 1983, he served with the National Multiple Sclerosis Society for 22 years where he was vice president for Research Programs. His responsibilities there included directing, evaluating and managing the world's largest private MS research and research training program (nearly $400 million in basic, clinical, and applied research) at a time when the first disease-modifying therapies for MS were developed, and he served the Society as a communicator and public spokesperson on scientific and clinical issues. Dr. Reingold has extensive consulting experience with industry, academic and foundation research programs, and has over 60 relevant professional publications.

Index